STUDY GUIDE

Anatomy & Physiology
Essentials

Publisher

The Goodheart-Willcox Company, Inc.

Tinley Park, IL

www.g-w.com

Contents

14 The Digestive System and Metabolism

15 The Urinary System

16 The Male and Female Reproductive Systems

NOTES

1 Foundations of Human Anatomy and Physiology

Name: _____   Date: _____

Section 1.1 Vocabulary Review

Match each vocabulary word with its definition.

A. abdominal cavity
B. abdominopelvic cavity
C. anatomical position
D. anatomy
E. anterior (ventral) cavity
F. cranial cavity
G. frontal plane
H. metric system
I. middle ear cavities
J. nasal cavity
K. oral cavity
L. orbital cavities
M. pelvic cavity
N. physiology
O. posterior (dorsal) cavity
P. sagittal plane
Q. spinal cavity
R. thoracic cavity
S. transverse plane

_____ 1. body cavity containing the mouth

_____ 2. portion of the ventral body cavity above the diaphragm

_____ 3. used for numerical quantities universally

_____ 4. position in which a person faces forward with palms facing anteriorly

_____ 5. the study of how structures in the body function

_____ 6. body cavities containing the eyes

_____ 7. divides the body into front and back portions

_____ 8. name for the body cavity that encompasses the entire area of the ventral body cavity below the diaphragm

_____ 9. large body cavity toward the back of the body

_____ 10. the more superior of the two body cavities below the diaphragm

_____ 11. body cavity containing the brain

_____ 12. study of the structures of the body

_____ 13. the more inferior of the two body cavities below the diaphragm

_____ 14. large body cavity toward the front of the body

_____ 15. divides the body into upper and lower portions

_____ 16. body cavities that help to amplify sound

_____ 17. cavity containing the spinal cord

_____ 18. divides the body into left and right portions

_____ 19. cavity behind the nose

Section 1.1 Study Questions

1. How can a frontal plane help you understand the body cavities?

2. Which body plane helps you visualize the terms *anterior* and *posterior*?

3. Which body plane helps you visualize the terms *superior* and *inferior*?

4. If a physician states that the patient has a cyst on the lateral aspect of the ovary, what does this mean?

5. What is the definition of a body cavity?

6. DNA testing can be done by taking a buccal swab. What part of the body does this involve?

7. What structure divides the ventral cavity into two smaller cavities?

8. In humans, what directional terms mean the same as *posterior* and *anterior*?

9. Why is it necessary to subdivide the abdominopelvic body cavity?

10. Why is the metric system used commonly around the world?

Section 1.1 Labeling
Abdominal Quadrants

Identify the correct location of each quadrant.

Labeling Terms

A. left lower quadrant
B. left upper quadrant
C. right lower quadrant
D. right upper quadrant

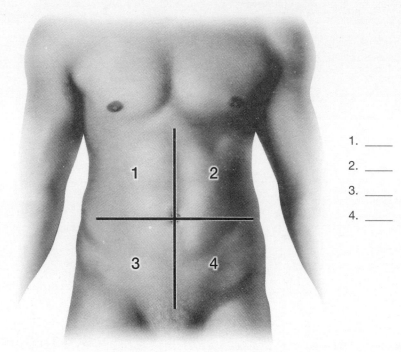

1. _____
2. _____
3. _____
4. _____

© Body Scientific International

Abdominal Regions

Identify the correct location of each abdominal region.

Labeling Terms

A. epigastric
B. hypogastric
C. left hypochondriac
D. left iliac
E. left lumbar
F. right hypochondriac
G. right iliac
H. right lumbar
I. umbilical

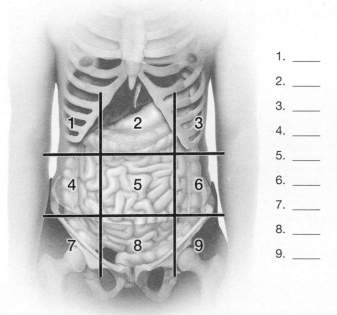

1. _____
2. _____
3. _____
4. _____
5. _____
6. _____
7. _____
8. _____
9. _____

© Body Scientific International

Name: _____   Date: _____

Body Cavities

Identify the correct location of each body cavity.

Labeling Terms

A. abdominal
B. abdominopelvic
C. anterior (ventral)
D. cranial

E. diaphragm
F. middle ear
G. nasal

H. oral
I. orbital
J. pelvic

K. posterior (dorsal)
L. spinal
M. thoracic

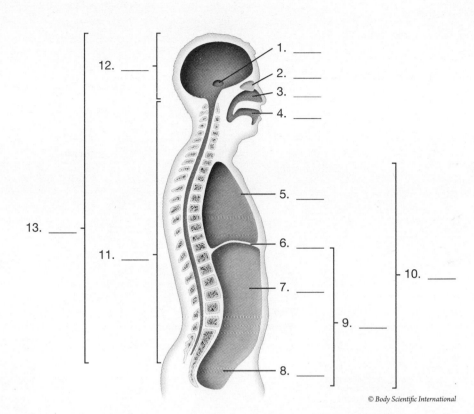

1. ____
2. ____
3. ____
4. ____
5. ____
6. ____
7. ____
8. ____
9. ____
10. ____
11. ____
12. ____
13. ____

© Body Scientific International

Section 1.2 Vocabulary Review

Match each vocabulary word with its definition.

A. atoms
B. cells
C. control center
D. effector
E. homeostasis
F. homeostatic imbalance
G. homeostatic mechanisms
H. metabolic rate
I. metabolism
J. molecules
K. negative feedback
L. organ
M. organ system
N. positive feedback
O. receptor
P. tissues

____ 1. body part that performs a specific function

____ 2. commands an action to an effector based on information received from sensory receptors

____ 3. groups of similar cells

____ 4. all necessary chemical reactions in the organism

____ 5. increases a condition that has exceeded the normal homeostatic range

____ 6. state in which the body is unable to keep the body's internal environment in the normal range

____ 7. particles that contain two or more atoms

____ 8. smallest building blocks of living things

____ 9. processes that maintain homeostasis

____ 10. transmitter that senses changes

____ 11. a group of organs working together

____ 12. the speed at which chemical reactions take place in the body

____ 13. tiny particles of matter

____ 14. unit that receives a command from the control center

____ 15. state of regulated physiological balance

____ 16. restoring homeostasis by reversing a condition that exceeds the normal range

Section 1.2 Study Questions

1. What is the basic building block of the human body?

2. What two organ systems control activities of the body, and by what mechanisms?

3. Which organ system filters extracellular fluids and returns them to the bloodstream?

4. Which two organ systems include the pancreas?

5. Name three organ systems that eliminate wastes.

6. Which two organ systems include the testes and ovaries?

7. Why is the term *homeostasis* considered one of the most important words in the study of anatomy and physiology?

8. Describe an example of a negative feedback system in the human body.

9. Describe an example of a positive feedback system in the human body.

10. Why does your metabolic rate influence your weight?

Section 1.2 Labeling: Organization of the Body

Identify each level of organization in the human body.

Labeling Terms

A. atom
B. body system
C. cell

D. molecule
E. organ
F. organelle

G. organism
H. tissue

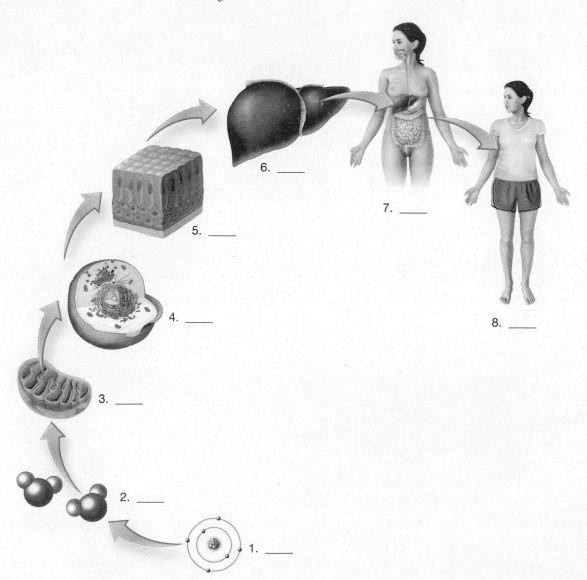

6. _____

7. _____

5. _____

4. _____

8. _____

3. _____

2. _____

1. _____

Name: _____   Date: _____

Section 1.3 Vocabulary Review

Match each vocabulary word with its definition.

A. bending
B. combined loading
C. compression
D. elastic
E. force
F. kinetics
G. mass
H. net force
I. plastic
J. pressure
K. shear
L. stress
M. tension
N. torque
O. torsion
P. weight

_____ 1. force distributed over a given area

_____ 2. loading pattern created by off-center forces

_____ 3. force equal to gravitational acceleration exerted on an object's mass

_____ 4. force that acts along a surface at a perpendicular angle

_____ 5. simultaneous action of two or more types of forces

_____ 6. quantity of matter contained in an object

_____ 7. force resulting from the summation of forces acting on a body

_____ 8. structure returns to its original size and shape after the application of a force

_____ 9. pulling force on a structure

_____ 10. study that analyzes the action of forces

_____ 11. squeezing force applied to a structure

_____ 12. loading pattern that causes a structure to twist

_____ 13. push or pull acting on a structure

_____ 14. force distribution inside a structure

_____ 15. structure remains deformed after application of a force

_____ 16. rotary effect of a force

Section 1.3 Study Questions

1. Why is it useful to study kinetics?

2. What is the net force on an object?

3. Would the mass of an object vary on another planet?

4. Why might the weight of an object vary on another planet?

5. If you jump and land on your feet, what type of force results?

6. If you hang from a pull-up bar, what type of force results?

7. How do shear force and compression force differ?

8. If you slide into home base, what type of force results?

9. Contrast bending and combined loading.

10. What is the difference between an elastic and a plastic injury?

Section 1.3 Labeling
Three Directions of Stress

Identify the directions of stress.

Labeling terms

A. compression
B. original shape
C. shear
D. tension

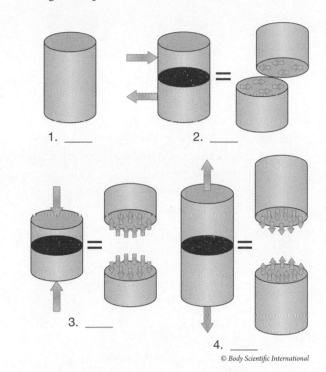

1. _____   2. _____

3. _____

4. _____

© Body Scientific International

Combined Loading

Identify the types of force distribution.

Labeling terms

A. bending
B. compression
C. tension
D. torsion

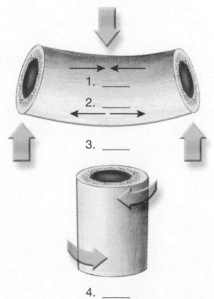

1. _____

2. _____

3. _____

4. _____

© Body Scientific International

Section 1.4 Vocabulary Review

Match each vocabulary word with its definition.

A. data
B. hypothesis
C. research question
D. science
E. scientific method
F. scientific theory
G. statistical inference
H. statistical significance

_____ 1. explanation based on tested and repeated, confirmed research

_____ 2. educated guess about the outcome of a study

_____ 3. systematic process to find solutions to problems

_____ 4. process that creates knowledge based on testable explanations and predictions

_____ 5. collected and recorded observations

_____ 6. generalizing the findings of a research study to a large population

_____ 7. question to be answered or problem to be solved

_____ 8. interpretation of data indicating that it can be generalized to the population represented in the study

Section 1.4 Study Questions

1. Why is it necessary to organize a scientific study?

2. What are data?

3. What is a hypothesis?

4. What condition is necessary in a research study in order to legitimately generalize conclusions from the data?

5. How do analyzing with statistical tools and drawing conclusions differ?

6. What is a scientific theory?

7. What were Galen's contributions to the study of the human body?

8. Which early anatomist discovered that the human heart has four chambers?

9. What was the contribution of William Harvey and Michael Servetus to anatomical understanding?

10. Who was the first scientist to use, view, and name cells?

Medical Terminology

For each item, identify the word parts and their meanings, and then provide the meaning of the medical term. Use a medical dictionary or the textbook if you need help.

1. abdominoplasty

    root/combining form: _____

    meaning: _____

    suffix: _____

    meaning: _____

    meaning of word: _____

2. cytology

    root/combining form: _____

    meaning: _____

    suffix: _____

    meaning: _____

    meaning of word: _____

3. dorsal

    root/combining form: _____

    meaning: _____

    suffix: _____

    meaning: _____

    meaning of word: _____

4. tonsillitis

    root/combining form: _____

    meaning: _____

    suffix: _____

    meaning: _____

    meaning of word: _____

5. leukemia

   root/combining form: _____

   meaning: _____

   suffix: _____

   meaning: _____

   meaning of word: _____

6. proctoscope

   root/combining form: _____

   meaning: _____

   suffix: _____

   meaning: _____

   meaning of word: _____

7. hypersecretion

   prefix: _____

   meaning: _____

   root/combining form: _____

   meaning: _____

   suffix: _____

   meaning: _____

   meaning of word: _____

8. hypothermic

   prefix: _____

   meaning: _____

   root/combining form: _____

   meaning: _____

   suffix: _____

   meaning: _____

   meaning of word: _____

9. endoscope

   root/combining form: _____

   meaning: _____

   suffix: _____

   meaning: _____

   meaning of word: _____

10. biology

   root/combining form: _____

   meaning: _____

   suffix: _____

   meaning: _____

   meaning of word: _____

NOTES

2 Molecules and Cells

Name: _____ Date: _____

Section 2.1 Vocabulary Review

Match each vocabulary word with its definition.

A. anion
B. atom
C. atomic number
D. cation
E. covalent bond
F. electron
G. element

H. hydrogen bond
I. ionic bond
J. ion
K. isotope
L. molecule
M. neutron
N. proton

_____ 1. determined by the number of protons

_____ 2. has the same number of protons, but a different number of neutrons

_____ 3. positively charged ion

_____ 4. negatively charged ion

_____ 5. type of bond that joins sodium chloride

_____ 6. type of bond that holds water together

_____ 7. a group of atoms bonded together

_____ 8. a combination of atoms of the same atomic number

_____ 9. any charged atom or molecule

_____ 10. negatively charged fundamental particle

_____ 11. positively charged fundamental particle

_____ 12. fundamental particle with no charge

_____ 13. bond that involves electron sharing

_____ 14. basic building block of matter

Section 2.1 Study Questions

1. What determines the atomic number of an atom?

2. What are the four most abundant elements in the human body?

3. What are the charges associated with electrons, neutrons, and protons?

4. How do covalent and ionic bonds differ?

5. What are ions?

6. How do anions and cations differ?

7. How are hydrogen bonds useful in the structure of DNA?

8. Carbon-12 and Carbon-14 are both isotopes of carbon. How do they differ?

9. Why can radioactive substances be harmful to the body?

10. How can radioactive substances be beneficial to your health?

Section 2.2 Vocabulary Review

Match each vocabulary word with its definition.

A. amino acids
B. base pairs
C. chromosomes
D. deoxyribonucleic acid (DNA)
E. enzyme
F. fatty acid
G. glucose
H. glycogen
I. human genome
J. lipids
K. nucleic acids
L. nucleotides
M. peptide
N. pH
O. phospholipids
P. polymer
Q. polypeptide
R. ribonucleic acid (RNA)
S. steroids
T. triglycerides

_____ 1. scale that delineates between acids and bases

_____ 2. type of lipid that has both hydrophilic and hydrophobic areas

_____ 3. protein that speeds up a reaction

_____ 4. consists of a glycerol head and three fatty acid tails

_____ 5. molecules such as DNA and RNA

_____ 6. small components that make up proteins

_____ 7. fats and oils

_____ 8. testosterone and estrogen

_____ 9. part of the side of the DNA ladder with one attached nitrogen base

_____ 10. form of stored glucose in animals

_____ 11. The complete DNA of a human

_____ 12. composed of many similar subunits

_____ 13. type of bond that joins amino acids

_____ 14. structures that contain the genetic material in the nucleus

_____ 15. a molecule made of a hydrocarbon chain with a carboxylic acid group at one end

_____ 16. polymer of nucleotides with the bases adenine, guanine, thymine, cytosine

_____ 17. polymer of nucleotides with the bases adenine, guanine, uracil, cytosine

_____ 18. complementary nucleic acid bases: A + T, C + G

_____ 19. example of a monosaccharide

_____ 20. very long string of amino acids

Section 2.2 Study Questions

1. What is another term for saccharides?

2. Describe the difference between a simple carbohydrate and a complex carbohydrate.

3. Describe the four levels of protein structure.

4. What is an enzyme and how does it benefit a reaction?

5. Describe the structure of a triglyceride.

6. What are the three basic parts of a nucleotide?

7. What are the three differences between DNA and RNA?

8. Name the four main types of RNA and their individual functions.

9. How are hydrogen bonds advantageous to water molecules?

10. Describe the pH scale.

Section 2.2 Labeling: Levels of Protein Structure

Identify the levels of protein structure.

Labeling Terms

A. helix
B. pleated sheet

C. primary structure
D. quaternary structure

E. secondary structure
F. tertiary structure

1. _____

2. _____

3. _____   4. _____   5. _____   6. _____

© Body Scientific International

Section 2.3 Vocabulary Review

Match each vocabulary word with its definition.

A. active transport
B. adenosine triphosphate (ATP)
C. anticodon
D. centrioles
E. channel proteins
F. cilia
G. codon
H. cytokinesis
I. cytoplasm

J. cytoskeleton
K. endoplasmic reticulum (ER)
L. extracellular fluid
M. extracellular matrix
N. glycoproteins
O. Golgi apparatus
P. messenger RNA (mRNA)
Q. microvilli
R. mitochondria

S. mitosis
T. nucleus
U. passive transport
V. plasma membrane
W. ribosomes
X. RNA polymerase
Y. transcription
Z. transfer RNA (tRNA)

_____ 1. helps assemble amino acids into polypeptides

_____ 2. division of the cytoplasm

_____ 3. organelle that can be classified as smooth or rough

_____ 4. molecular form of energy

_____ 5. copies the recipe in the nucleus and takes it to the ribosome in protein synthesis

_____ 6. fluid outside of cells

_____ 7. cylinders of microtubules that aid in mitosis

_____ 8. three bases that code for an amino acid in DNA or RNA

_____ 9. three bases on tRNA that are complementary to those on mRNA

_____ 10. organelle that makes proteins

_____ 11. process by which nuclear material is split into two separate nuclei

_____ 12. watery, gel-like material in which cellular organelles are suspended

_____ 13. movement of a substance from a low concentration to a high concentration

_____ 14. proteins with attached carbohydrate groups

_____ 15. fluids are moved via these hair-like projections

_____ 16. solid or gel material that surrounds a cell

_____ 17. production of RNA from DNA

_____ 18. the "skin" of a cell

_____ 19. network of proteins that give support to the cell

_____ 20. enzyme that makes an RNA molecule complementary to DNA

_____ 21. proteins with a hollow center that allow access into or out of a cell

_____ 22. modifies and packages proteins

_____ 23. organelle that produces ATP

_____ 24. tiny finger-like projections that increase surface area

_____ 25. movement of a substance from a high concentration to a low concentration

_____ 26. portion of a cell containing DNA

Section 2.3 Study Questions

1. Describe the structure of the plasma membrane.

2. What is the primary difference between passive and active processes?

3. What are the functions of ribosomes, the Golgi apparatus, and mitochondria?

4. Describe the roles of the nucleus and the nucleolus.

5. What is the function of DNA in protein synthesis?

6. In one sentence, describe the function of mRNA in protein synthesis.

7. Describe what is meant by the terms *codon* and *anticodon*.

8. In simple terms, what is the function of tRNA in protein synthesis?

9. Describe the events that occur in interphase.

10. What is the difference between mitosis and cytokinesis?

Section 2.3 Labeling
Parts of a Cell

Identify the parts of a cell.

Labeling Terms

A. centrosome
B. cytoplasm
C. cytoskeleton
D. Golgi apparatus

E. lysosome
F. mitochondrion
G. nucleus
H. peroxisome

I. plasma membrane
J. ribosome
K. rough endoplasmic reticulum
L. smooth endoplasmic reticulum

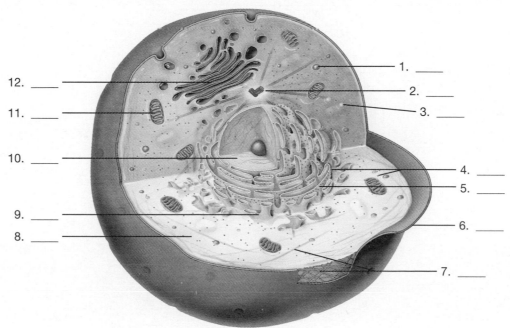

1. _____
2. _____
3. _____
4. _____
5. _____
6. _____
7. _____
8. _____
9. _____
10. _____
11. _____
12. _____

© *Body Scientific International*

Plasma Membrane Structure

Identify the structures of the plasma membrane.

Labeling Terms

A. carbohydrate group
B. cytoplasm
C. extracellular matrix
D. glycoprotein

E. ion channel protein
F. membrane pump protein
G. microfilament

H. peripheral protein
I. structural protein (integrin)
J. transmembrane proteins

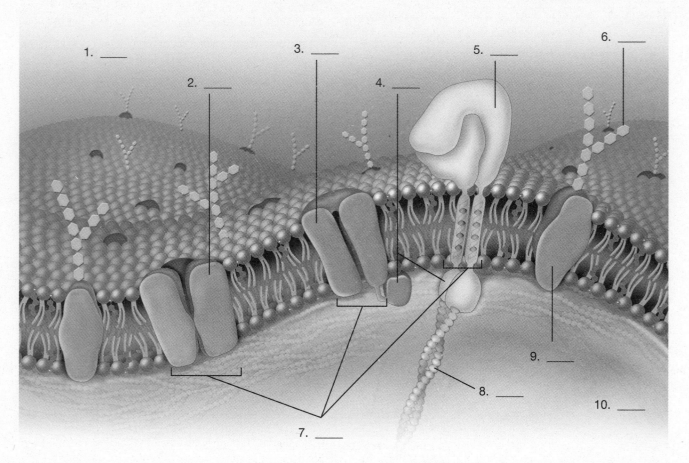

1. ____ 2. ____ 3. ____ 4. ____ 5. ____ 6. ____ 7. ____ 8. ____ 9. ____ 10. ____

© Body Scientific International

Nucleus and Endoplasmic Reticulum

Identify the components of the nucleus and endoplasmic reticulum.

Labeling Terms

A. chromatin
B. cisternae
C. nuclear envelope
D. nucleolus
E. ribosomes
F. rough endoplasmic reticulum
G. smooth endoplasmic reticulum

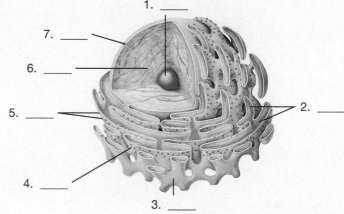

1. ____ 7. ____ 6. ____ 5. ____ 4. ____ 3. ____ 2. ____

© Body Scientific International

Medical Terminology

For each item, identify the word parts and their meanings, and then provide the meaning of the medical term. Use a medical dictionary or the textbook if you need help.

1. somnambulist

    root/combining form: _____

    meaning: _____

    root/combining form: _____

    meaning: _____

    suffix: _____

    meaning: _____

    meaning of word: _____

2. thermometer

    root/combining form: _____

    meaning: _____

    suffix: _____

    meaning: _____

    meaning of word: _____

3. mitotic

    root/combining form: _____

    meaning: _____

    suffix: _____

    meaning: _____

    meaning of word: _____

4. carcinogenic

    root/combining form: _____

    meaning: _____

    root/combining form: _____

    meaning: _____

    suffix: _____

    meaning: _____

    meaning of word: _____

5. glucometer

    root/combining form: _____

    meaning: _____

    suffix: _____

    meaning: _____

    meaning of word: _____

6. toxoid

    root/combining form: _____

    meaning: _____

    suffix: _____

    meaning: _____

    meaning of word: _____

7. deoxyglucose

    prefix: _____

    meaning: _____

    prefix: _____

    meaning: _____

    root/combining form: _____

    meaning: _____

    meaning of word: _____

8. adipometer

    root/combining form: _____

    meaning: _____

    suffix: _____

    meaning: _____

    meaning of word: _____

9. phosphoric

    root/combining form: _____

    meaning: _____

    suffix: _____

    meaning: _____

    meaning of word: _____

10. carcinoid

    root/combining form: _____

    meaning: _____

    suffix: _____

    meaning: _____

    meaning of word: _____

3 Body Tissues

Name: _____ Date: _____

Section 3.1 Vocabulary Review

Match each vocabulary word with its definition.

A. connective tissue
B. ectoderm
C. endoderm
D. epithelial tissue
E. extracellular matrix
F. histology
G. mesoderm
H. muscle tissue
I. nerve tissue

_____ 1. embryonic tissue that becomes lining of the lungs and gastrointestinal tract

_____ 2. the study of tissues

_____ 3. category that includes bone, blood, and cartilage

_____ 4. embryonic tissue that becomes nervous tissue

_____ 5. composed of neurons and glial cells

_____ 6. classified as skeletal, smooth, or cardiac

_____ 7. embryonic tissue that becomes connective and muscle tissue

_____ 8. category that covers external and some internal areas of the body

_____ 9. material between cells in tissues

Section 3.1 Study Questions

1. Which category of tissues forms barriers between the body and the external environment?

2. What are some functions of connective tissue?

3. What are some functions of muscle tissue?

4. What are some functions of nerve tissue?

5. Which type of tissue is derived from all three types of embryonic layers?

6. Which types of tissue are derived from endoderm?

7. Which types of tissue are derived from mesoderm?

8. Which types of tissue are derived from ectoderm?

9. What causes the disease spina bifida?

10. Why is the study of pathology so important?

Section 3.1 Labeling: Identification of Tissue Types

Identify each type of tissue.

Labeling terms

A. connective tissue
B. epithelial tissue
C. muscle tissue
D. nerve tissue

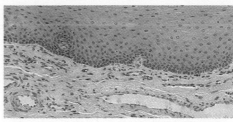

Jose Luis Calvo/Shutterstock.com

1. _____

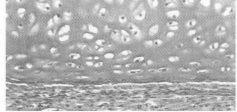

Anna Jurkovska/Shutterstock.com

2. _____

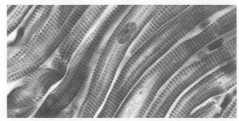

Jose Luis Calvo/Shutterstock.com

3. _____

Kateryna Kon/Shutterstock.com

4. _____

Section 3.2 Vocabulary Review

Match each vocabulary word with its definition.

A. cardiac muscle
B. cartilage
C. chondroblasts
D. compressive strength
E. elasticity
F. endocrine gland
G. exocrine gland
H. glands
I. lumen
J. neurons
K. osseous tissue
L. simple epithelia
M. skeletal muscle
N. smooth muscle
O. stratified epithelia
P. tensile strength

_____ 1. the area within a tube

_____ 2. bone

_____ 3. type of muscle surrounding organs

_____ 4. ability to withstand an inward-pressing force
without buckling

_____ 5. form cartilage

_____ 6. voluntary muscle that is usually attached to bone

_____ 7. gland that secretes through ductwork to outside
the body

_____ 8. ability to withstand an outward-pulling force
without tearing

_____ 9. muscle found only in the heart

_____ 10. characteristic of material that regains its original
shape after stretching

_____ 11. gland without ductwork that secretes into
extracellular space

_____ 12. cells that receive and send messages to areas
of the body

_____ 13. single layer of epithelial cells

_____ 14. many layers of epithelial cells

_____ 15. cells that form and secrete substances

_____ 16. type of connective tissue that is very flexible

Section 3.2 Study Questions

1. What is the difference between simple epithelia
and stratified epithelia?

2. Describe the three shapes of epithelial cells.

3. What are the differences between exocrine and endocrine
glands?

4. What is the criterion for categorizing exocrine glands?

5. Describe the extracellular matrix in blood. How is this
different from the matrices of other connective tissue?

6. Where in the body is reticular connective tissue found?

7. What are the functions and locations of the three types
of cartilage?

8. What is the purpose of osseous tissue?

9. Describe the three types of muscle.

10. What nerves comprise the peripheral nervous system?

Section 3.2 Labeling
Types of Epithelia

Identify the types of epithelia.

Labeling Terms

A. columnar
B. cuboidal
C. simple
D. squamous
E. stratified

© Body Scientific International

Exocrine Gland Structure

Identify the structures of the exocrine gland.

Labeling Terms

A. alveolar (spherical) shaped
B. compound alveolar
C. compound tubular

D. compound tubuloalveolar
(both tubular and aveolar shaped)
E. duct

F. secretory unit
G. surface of epithelium
H. tubular shaped

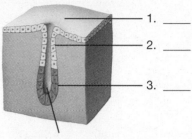

1. _____
2. _____
3. _____

4. _____

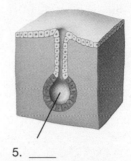

5. _____

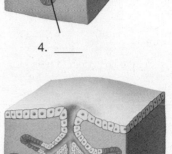

6. _____

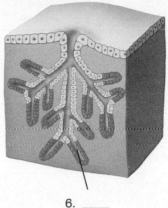

7. _____

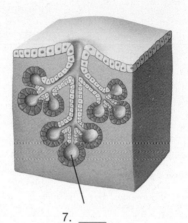

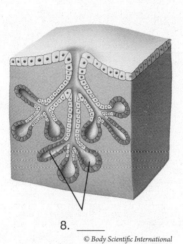

8. _____

© Body Scientific International

Section 3.3 Vocabulary Review

Match each vocabulary word with its definition.

A. biopsy
B. carcinoma
C. cystic fibrosis
D. eczema
E. leukemia
F. lymphoma
G. Marfan syndrome
H. sarcoma
I. systemic lupus erythematosus

_____ 1. autoimmune disease that affects connective tissue
_____ 2. causes immature white blood cells to be created
_____ 3. cancer of lymphatic tissue
_____ 4. produces thick mucus causing respiratory and digestive issues
_____ 5. cancer that originates in epithelial tissue
_____ 6. cancer that originates in connective tissue
_____ 7. microscopic examination of body tissue
_____ 8. characteristics include being tall with long fingers, toes, arms, and legs
_____ 9. also known as *atopic dermatitis*

Section 3.3 Study Questions

1. In what type of tissue does eczema originate?
2. What causes eczema?
3. Which disease results from defective CFTR genes?
4. What two organ systems are affected by cystic fibrosis?
5. How might you identify someone with Marfan syndrome?
6. Name the symptoms of systemic lupus erythematosus.
7. What is the difference between a carcinoma and a sarcoma?
8. Differentiate between leukemia and lymphoma.
9. What are the four most common types of cancer in the United States?
10. Where in the body do most carcinomas originate?

Medical Terminology

For each item, identify the word parts and their meanings, and then provide the meaning of the medical term. Use a medical dictionary or the textbook if you need help.

1. osteoporosis

   root/combining form: _____

   meaning: _____

   root/combining form: _____

   meaning: _____

   suffix: _____

   meaning: _____

   meaning of word: _____

2. ossification

   root/combining form: _____

   meaning: _____

   suffix: _____

   meaning: _____

   meaning of word: _____

3. neuralgia

   root/combining form: _____

   meaning: _____

   suffix: _____

   meaning: _____

   meaning of word: _____

4. ophthalmology

   root/combining form: _____

   meaning: _____

   suffix: _____

   meaning: _____

   meaning of word: _____

5. erythroblast

   root/combining form: _____

   meaning: _____

   root/combining form: _____

   meaning: _____

   meaning of word: _____

6. hemocytoblast

   root/combining form: _____

   meaning: _____

   root/combining form: _____

   meaning: _____

   root/combining form: _____

   meaning: _____

   meaning of word: _____

7. blastoma

   root/combining form: _____

   meaning: _____

   suffix: _____

   meaning: _____

   meaning of word: _____

8. dermatitis

   root/combining form: _____

   meaning: _____

   suffix: _____

   meaning: _____

   meaning of word: _____

9. dermopathy

   root/combining form: _____

   meaning: _____

   suffix: _____

   meaning: _____

   meaning of word: _____

Name: _____   Date: _____

10. ectopic

   prefix: _____

   meaning: _____

   suffix: _____

   meaning: _____

   meaning of word: _____

NOTES

4 Membranes and the Integumentary System

Name: _____   Date: _____

Section 4.1 Vocabulary Review

Match each vocabulary word with its definition.

A. cutaneous membrane
B. epithelial membranes
C. membranes
D. mucous membranes
E. pericardium
F. peritoneum
G. pleura
H. serous fluid
I. serous membranes
J. synovial fluid
K. synovial membrane

_____ 1. membrane surrounding the heart
_____ 2. lubricating fluid to reduce friction between membranes
_____ 3. lubricating fluid found in joints
_____ 4. skin
_____ 5. membrane lining the abdominal cavity
_____ 6. produces lubricating fluid in joints
_____ 7. membrane surrounding the lungs
_____ 8. membranes open to the outside world
_____ 9. coverings of external and internal body surfaces
_____ 10. thin layers of tissue
_____ 11. membranes lining areas closed to the outside world

Section 4.1 Study Questions

1. What is the function of membranes?
2. Describe the structure of a mucous membrane.
3. Where in the body would you find the lamina propria?
4. How do mucous membranes protect the body?
5. How do mucous membranes and serous membranes differ?
6. What organs are associated with the pericardium and pleura?

7. In reference to serous membranes, define the terms *visceral* and *parietal*.
8. What is the lubricating fluid in serous membranes and where is it produced?
9. What is a bursa?
10. What is the lubricating fluid in synovial joints and where is it produced?

Section 4.1 Labeling

Synovial Joint

Identify the structures in and around the synovial joint.

Labeling Terms

A. articular capsule
B. articular cartilage
C. junction of membrane with cartilage
D. lateral meniscus
E. medial meniscus
F. patella
G. synovial membrane

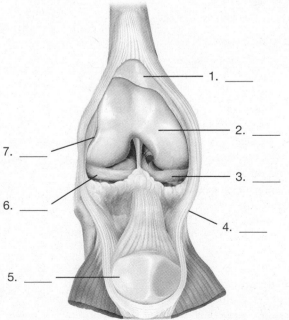

© Body Scientific International

Name: _____ Date: _____

Section 4.2 Vocabulary Review

Match each vocabulary word with its definition.

A. dermis
B. epidermal dendritic cells
C. epidermis
D. hypodermis
E. integumentary system
F. keratin
G. keratinocytes
H. melanin
I. melanocytes
J. Merkel cells

K. papillary layer
L. reticular layer
M. sebaceous glands
N. sebum
O. stratum basale
P. stratum corneum
Q. stratum granulosum
R. stratum lucidum
S. stratum spinosum
T. sudoriferous glands

_____ 1. pigment in the skin
_____ 2. substance released from oil glands
_____ 3. youngest epidermal layer
_____ 4. touch receptors
_____ 5. subcutaneous fascia
_____ 6. cells producing pigment
_____ 7. found only in thick-skinned areas of the body
_____ 8. superficial layer of the dermis
_____ 9. protein that adds strength to tissue
_____ 10. epidermal layer between stratum spinosum and stratum lucidum
_____ 11. layer of oldest epidermal cells
_____ 12. cells that produce a substance that adds strength to skin
_____ 13. outer main layer of skin
_____ 14. organ system that includes skin
_____ 15. main skin layer between the epidermis and hypodermis
_____ 16. cells in skin that produce the immune response
_____ 17. deep layer of the dermis
_____ 18. oil glands
_____ 19. sweat glands
_____ 20. epidermal layer between stratum basale and stratum granulosum

Section 4.2 Study Questions

1. What clues can the following alternative skin colors and hues give about your health: yellow, pale, red, orange, and blue?
2. What is the difference between eccrine glands and apocrine glands?
3. Describe the cell layers of the epidermis.
4. Where in the body would you find a lunule?
5. What causes goose bumps?
6. What are the two layers of the dermis?
7. What are the functions of epidermal dendritic cells and Merkel cells?
8. Which vitamin is manufactured in the skin, and under what condition?
9. Which type of cell comprises the majority of the epidermis?
10. What are the functions of the hypodermis?

Section 4.2 Labeling
Skin Section

Identify the structures of the skin.

Labeling Terms

A. arrector pili muscle
B. artery
C. dermis
D. epidermis
E. hair follicle
F. hair shaft
G. hypodermis
H. lamellar corpuscle
I. lipocytes (fat cells)
J. nerve fibers
K. papillary layer
L. pore of sweat gland duct
M. reticular layer
N. sebaceous gland
O. sweat gland
P. sweat gland duct
Q. tactile corpuscle
R. vein

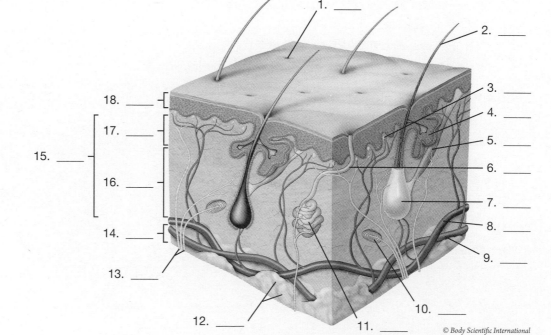

© Body Scientific International

Layers of the Epidermis

Identify the layers of the epidermis.

Labeling Terms

A. dermis
B. stratum basale
C. stratum corneum
D. stratum granulosum
E. stratum lucidum
F. stratum spinosum

1. _____
2. _____
3. _____
4. _____
5. _____
6. _____

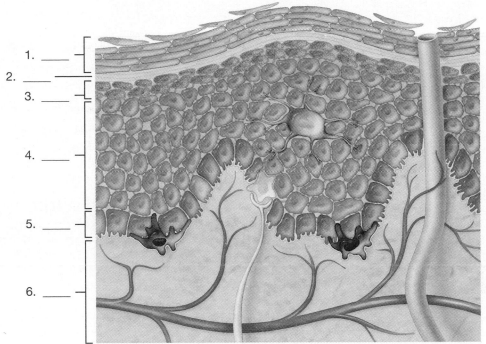

© Body Scientific International

Eccrine and Apocrine Glands

Identify the eccrine and apocrine glands.

Labeling Terms

A. apocrine sweat gland
B. cells of epidermis
C. dermis
D. eccrine sweat gland
E. follicle and root
F. hair strand
G. sebaceous gland
H. stratum corneum

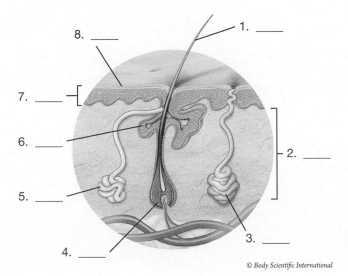

8. _____
7. _____
6. _____
5. _____
4. _____
1. _____
2. _____
3. _____

© Body Scientific International

Base of a Hair Follicle

Identify the base of a hair follicle.

Labeling Terms

A. connective tissue papilla
B. dermal sheath
C. epidermal sheath
D. hair follicle
E. hair strand
F. lipocytes
G. melanocyte
H. matrix

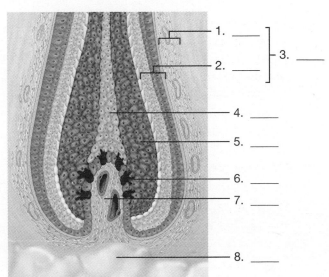

1. _____
2. _____
3. _____
4. _____
5. _____
6. _____
7. _____
8. _____

© Body Scientific International

Section 4.3 Vocabulary Review

Match each vocabulary word with its definition.

A. basal cell carcinoma
B. cellulitis
C. common warts
D. first-degree burns
E. fourth-degree burns
F. herpes simplex virus type 1 (HSV-1)
G. herpes simplex virus type 2 (HSV-2)
H. herpes varicella
I. herpes zoster
J. impetigo
K. malignant melanoma
L. peritonitis
M. plantar warts
N. pleurisy
O. psoriasis
P. rule of nines
Q. second-degree burns
R. squamous cell carcinoma
S. third-degree burns
T. tinea

_____   1. most common type of skin cancer

_____   2. inflamed peritoneum

_____   3. common viral childhood disease

_____   4. causes cold sores

_____   5. burn that causes skin to blister

_____   6. fungal infection

_____   7. growths that occur on hands and feet and often disappear

_____   8. method to determine the extent of a burn

_____   9. burn that affects not only the skin, but also tissues below

_____ 10. inflammation of the membranes surrounding the lungs

_____ 11. most dangerous form of skin cancer

_____ 12. burn that destroys all the layers of the skin

_____ 13. bacterial infection of the skin that results in bumps on the faces of young children

_____ 14. a dormant virus that appears in adulthood after a child has chickenpox

_____ 15. genital form of a virus

_____ 16. bacterial infection of the skin that presents as a red, painful area

_____ 17. burn that affects only the epidermis

_____ 18. skin disease that causes flaky, itchy skin

_____ 19. bumps on the feet that grow inward

_____ 20. a type of skin cancer that looks red and scaly

Section 4.3 Study Questions

1. What is the purpose of the rule of nines?
2. Explain the ABCD rule for identifying a malignant melanoma.
3. What is the main difference between herpes simplex virus type 1 and type 2?
4. How do common warts and plantar warts differ?
5. Where on the body would you find a tinea cruris infection?
6. How are pleurisy and peritonitis alike? How do they differ?
7. What is the cause of decubitus ulcers?
8. Describe the four categories of burns.
9. What is the danger associated with high-risk HPV infections?
10. What is cellulitis?

Medical Terminology

For each item, identify the word parts and their meanings, and then provide the meaning of the medical term. Use a medical dictionary or the textbook if you need help.

1. cytogenetics

    root/combining form: _____

    meaning: _____

    root/combining form: _____

    meaning: _____

    suffix: _____

    meaning: _____

    meaning of word: _____

2. dermabrasion

    root/combining form: _____

    meaning: _____

    root/combining form: _____

    meaning: _____

    suffix: _____

    meaning: _____

    meaning of word: _____

3. bronchiole

    root/combining form: _____

    meaning: _____

    suffix: _____

    meaning: _____

    meaning of word: _____

4. cutaneovisceral

    root/combining form: _____

    meaning: _____

    root/combining form: _____

    meaning: _____

    suffix: _____

    meaning: _____

    meaning of word: _____

5. dermatomyosis

    root/combining form: _____

    meaning: _____

    root/combining form: _____

    meaning: _____

    suffix: _____

    meaning: _____

    meaning of word: _____

6. epicranial

    prefix: _____

    meaning: _____

    root/combining form: _____

    meaning: _____

    suffix: _____

    meaning: _____

    meaning of word: _____

7. perigastric

    prefix: _____

    meaning: _____

    root/combining form: _____

    meaning: _____

    suffix: _____

    meaning: _____

    meaning of word: _____

8. gastroesophageal

    root/combining form: _____

    meaning: _____

    root/combining form: _____

    meaning: _____

    suffix: _____

    meaning: _____

    meaning of word: _____

9. bronchopathy

    root/combining form: _____

    meaning: _____

    suffix: _____

    meaning: _____

    meaning of word: _____

10. perimysium

    prefix: _____

    meaning: _____

    root/combining form: _____

    meaning: _____

    suffix: _____

    meaning: _____

    meaning of word: _____

NOTES

5 The Skeletal System

Name: _____ Date: _____

Section 5.1 Vocabulary Review

Match each vocabulary word with its definition.

A. appositional growth
B. articular cartilage
C. bone marrow
D. cortical bone
E. diaphysis
F. epiphyseal plate
G. epiphysis
H. Haversian canals
I. Haversian system
J. hematopoiesis
K. medullary cavity
L. ossification
M. osteoblasts
N. osteoclasts
O. osteocytes
P. osteons
Q. perforating (Volkmann's) canals
R. periosteum
S. remodeling
T. Sharpey's fibers
U. trabecular bone

_____ 1. growth plate

_____ 2. cavity in the center of a long bone

_____ 3. mature bone cells

_____ 4. spongy bone

_____ 5. red or yellow material within a long bone

_____ 6. attach the periosteum to the bone

_____ 7. compact bone

_____ 8. making bone

_____ 9. making blood cells

_____ 10. cells that break down bone

_____ 11. adding new layers to bone

_____ 12. membrane attached to the outside of a long bone

_____ 13. shaft of a long bone

_____ 14. another name for an osteon

_____ 15. cells that build bone

_____ 16. structures perpendicular to Haversian canals

_____ 17. end of a long bone

_____ 18. process in which osteoclasts and osteoblasts are active

_____ 19. cartilage covering the ends of bone

_____ 20. contains concentric lamellae

_____ 21. runs lengthwise down the middle of an osteon

Section 5.1 Study Questions

1. What are the main components of bone?

2. Name and describe the two types of bone marrow.

3. What are the advantages of cortical bone and trabecular bone?

4. What are the five basic shapes of bones?

5. Where are the periosteum and endosteum located in a long bone?

6. How does the arrangement of Haversian canals and perforating (Volkmann's) canals differ?

7. Describe the process of bone remodeling.

8. Explain the process of longitudinal bone growth.

9. How does appositional growth occur?

10. What is the relationship between parathyroid hormone and calcitonin?

Section 5.1 Labeling
Categories of Bone

Identify the shape categories of bone.

Labeling Terms

A. flat bone
B. irregular bones
C. long bone
D. sesamoid bone
E. short bones

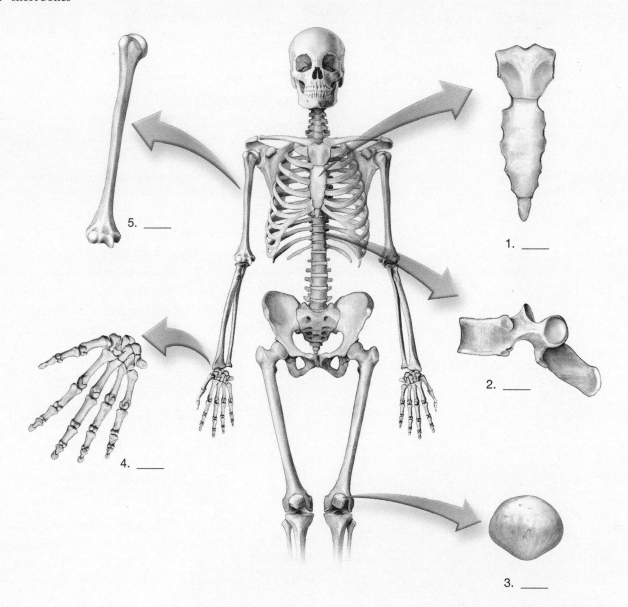

5. ____

1. ____

2. ____

4. ____

3. ____

© Body Scientific International

Name: _____ Date: _____

Parts of a Long Bone

Identify the parts of a long bone.

Labeling Terms

A. articular cartilage
B. blood vessel
C. cortical bone
D. diaphysis
E. endosteum
F. epiphysis

G. medullary canal
H. periosteum
I. red marrow cavities
J. trabecular bone
K. yellow bone marrow

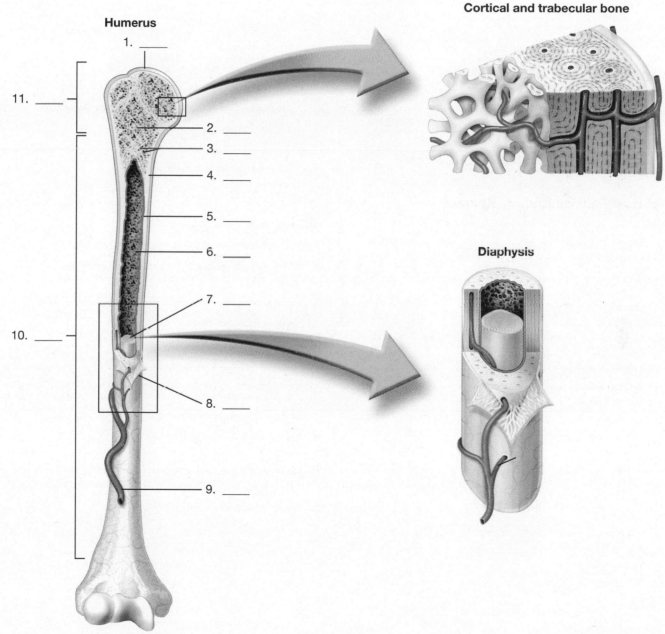

Humerus

1. ____

11. ____

2. ____

3. ____

4. ____

5. ____

6. ____

7. ____

10. ____

8. ____

9. ____

Cortical and trabecular bone

Diaphysis

© *Body Scientific International*

Cross Section of a Long Bone

Identify the cross section of a long bone.

Labeling Terms

A. cortical bone
B. endosteum
C. medullary cavity
D. osteoblast activity
E. osteoclast activity
F. periosteum

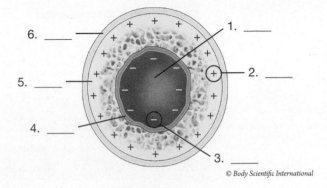

© Body Scientific International

Section 5.2 Vocabulary Review

Match each vocabulary word with its definition.

A. atlas
B. axial skeleton
C. axis
D. cervical region
E. coccyx
F. cranium
G. facial bones
H. fontanel
I. intervertebral discs
J. lumbar region
K. mandible
L. maxillary bones
M. median sacral crest
N. sacral canal
O. sacral hiatus
P. sacrum
Q. skull
R. sternum
S. sutures
T. thoracic cage
U. thoracic region
V. vertebra

_____ 1. joints between cranial bones

_____ 2. tailbone

_____ 3. bones of the upper jaw

_____ 4. segment of the backbone

_____ 5. C2

_____ 6. soft spot in a baby's skull

_____ 7. breastbone

_____ 8. C1 – C7

_____ 9. located between the vertebral bodies

_____ 10. structure superior to the coccyx

_____ 11. consists of 14 bones

_____ 12. L1 – L5

_____ 13. consists of ribs, sternum, and thoracic vertebrae

_____ 14. C1

_____ 15. fused spinous processes of superior sacral vertebrae

_____ 16. skull, spine, thoracic cage

_____ 17. T1 – T12

_____ 18. term for fused bones at the back of the head

_____ 19. lower jaw

_____ 20. bones of the head

_____ 21. vertebral canal in the sacrum

_____ 22. opening in inferior end of sacrum canal

Section 5.2 Study Questions

1. Which bones constitute the axial skeleton?

2. What are fontanels, and how are they advantageous to an infant?

3. What are the locations of the four sutures in the skull?

4. What are the names and locations of the eight cranial bones?

5. Which bone is the only movable cranial or facial bone?

6. Describe the joint between the atlas and the axis.

7. Describe the regions of the spine.

8. Where does the spinal cord pass through each vertebra?

9. Name and describe three abnormal curvatures of the spine.

10. Name the three categories of ribs.

Section 5.2 Labeling
The Skeleton
Identify the major bones of the axial and appendicular skeleton.

Labeling Terms

A. calcaneous
B. carpals
C. clavicle
D. coccyx
E. coxal (hip) bone
F. cranium
G. facial bones
H. femur
I. fibula
J. humerus
K. metacarpals
L. metatarsals
M. patella
N. phalanges of the feet
O. phalanges of the hands
P. radius
Q. ribs
R. sacrum
S. scapula
T. skull
U. sternum
V. tarsals
W. thoracic cage
X. tibia
Y. ulna
Z. vertebral
   column (spine)

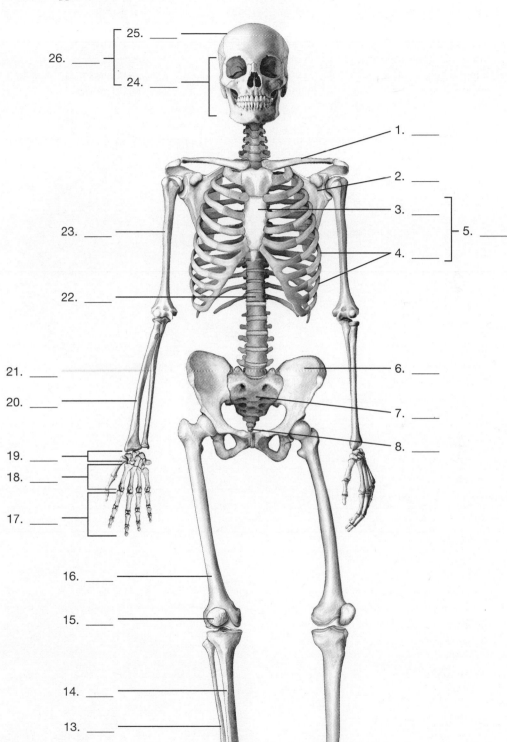

© Body Scientific International

Lateral View of the Skull

Identify the bones of the skull.

Labeling Terms

A. alveolar processes
B. coronal suture
C. ethmoid bone
D. external acoustic meatus
E. frontal bone
F. lacrimal bone

G. lambdoid suture
H. mandible (body)
I. mandibular ramus
J. mastoid process
K. maxilla
L. mental foreman

M. nasal bone
N. occipital bone
O. parietal bone
P. sphenoid bone
Q. squamous suture
R. styloid process

S. temporal bone
T. zygomatic bone
U. zygomatic process

Lateral view

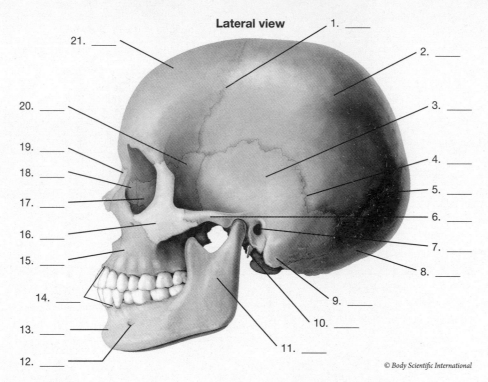

21. ____
20. ____
19. ____
18. ____
17. ____
16. ____
15. ____
14. ____
13. ____
12. ____

1. ____
2. ____
3. ____
4. ____
5. ____
6. ____
7. ____
8. ____
9. ____
10. ____
11. ____

© Body Scientific International

Anterior View of the Skull

Identify the bones of the skull.

Anterior view

Labeling Terms

A. alveolar processes
B. coronal suture
C. ethmoid bone
D. frontal bone
E. inferior nasal concha
F. lacrimal bone
G. mandible
H. mastoid process
I. maxilla
J. middle nasal concha
   of ethmoid bone
K. nasal bone
L. optic canal
M. parietal bone
N. sphenoid bone
O. superior orbital fissure
P. temporal bone
Q. vomer
R. zygomatic bone

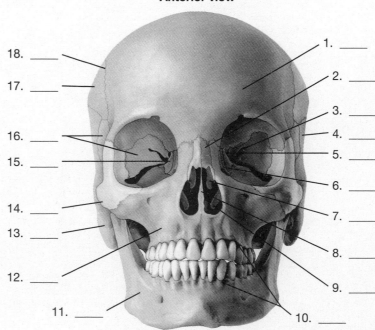

18. ____
17. ____
16. ____
15. ____
14. ____
13. ____
12. ____
11. ____

1. ____
2. ____
3. ____
4. ____
5. ____
6. ____
7. ____
8. ____
9. ____
10. ____

© Body Scientific International

The Vertebral Column

Identify the regions and curves of the vertebral column.

Labeling Terms

A. cervical curve
B. cervical region
C. coccyx
D. lumbar curve
E. lumbar region
F. sacral curve
G. sacrum
H. thoracic curve
I. thoracic region

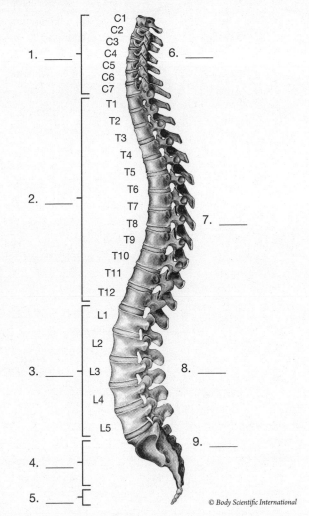

1. ____
2. ____
3. ____
4. ____
5. ____
6. ____
7. ____
8. ____
9. ____

C1 C2 C3 C4 C5 C6 C7
T1 T2 T3 T4 T5 T6 T7 T8 T9 T10 T11 T12
L1 L2 L3 L4 L5

© Body Scientific International

The Thoracic Cage

Identify the parts of the thoracic cage.

Labeling Terms

A. body
B. clavicle
C. costal cartilage
D. false ribs
E. floating ribs
F. jugular notch
G. manubrium
H. sternal angle
I. sternum
J. true ribs
K. xiphisternal joint
L. xiphoid process

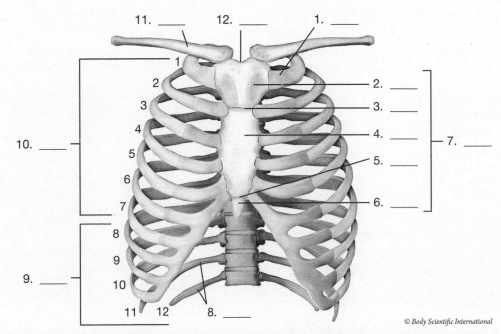

1. ____
2. ____
3. ____
4. ____
5. ____
6. ____
7. ____
8. ____
9. ____
10. ____
11. ____
12. ____

© Body Scientific International

Name: _____   Date: _____

Section 5.3 Vocabulary Review

Match each vocabulary word with its definition.

A. appendicular skeleton
B. calcaneus
C. carpal bones
D. clavicle
E. false pelvis
F. femur
G. fibula
H. humerus
I. lower extremity
J. metacarpal bones
K. metatarsal bones
L. patella
M. pectoral girdle
N. pelvis
O. phalanges
P. radius
Q. scapula
R. shoulder complex
S. tarsal bones
T. tibia
U. true pelvis
V. ulna
W. upper extremity

_____ 1. collarbone

_____ 2. includes the acromioclavicular, sternoclavicular, and glenohumeral joints

_____ 3. prominent bone in the lower leg

_____ 4. heel bone

_____ 5. bone of the upper arm

_____ 6. kneecap

_____ 7. finger and toe bones

_____ 8. shoulders, arms, and hands

_____ 9. bones of the arms and legs

_____ 10. ankle bones

_____ 11. bony portion of the pelvis superior to the pelvic inlet

_____ 12. clavicle and scapula

_____ 13. pelvis area surrounding the pelvic inlet

_____ 14. thigh bone

_____ 15. wrist bones

_____ 16. forearm bone on the thumb side

_____ 17. shoulder blade

_____ 18. includes bones of the pelvic girdle and coccyx

_____ 19. hips, legs, and feet

_____ 20. bones in between tarsals and phalanges

_____ 21. forearm bone on the little finger side

_____ 22. thinner bone in the lower leg

_____ 23. bones in between the carpals and phalanges

Section 5.3 Study Questions

1. Which bones constitute the appendicular skeleton?

2. Which joint in the shoulder complex attaches the clavicle to the torso?

3. Which portions of the elbow joint connect the humerus to the radius and ulna?

4. Which bones of the appendicular skeleton contain styloid processes?

5. What are the differences between a male and female pelvis?

6. Describe the hip joint.

7. Which bones articulate at the knee?

8. Which pairs of bones are joined by interosseous membranes?

9. In the extremities, which bones are classified as short bones?

10. How many phalanges are in the entire human body?

Section 5.3 Labeling
Anterior View of the Shoulder Girdle, Ribs, and Humerus

Identify the bones of the shoulder girdle, ribs, and humerus.

Labeling Terms

A. acromion
B. body of sternum
C. clavicle
D. corocoid process
E. costal cartilage
F. eighth rib
G. first rib
H. head of humerus
I. humerus
J. manubrium
K. scapula
L. seventh rib
M. sternoclavicular joint
N. twelfth thoracic vertebrae
O. xiphoid process

Anterior view

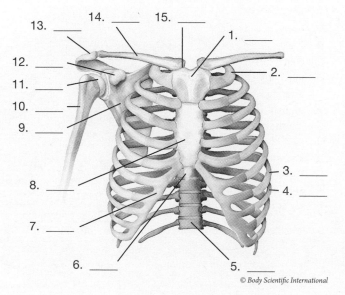

13. _____   14. _____   15. _____

1. _____

12. _____

2. _____

11. _____

10. _____

9. _____

8. _____

7. _____

3. _____

4. _____

6. _____   5. _____

© Body Scientific International

Anterior View of the Pelvis

Identify the bones of the pelvis.

Labeling Terms

A. acetabulum
B. coccyx
C. coxal bone

D. iliac crest
E. ilium
F. ischial spine

G. ischium
H. obturator foramen
I. pubic symphysis

J. pubis
K. sacroiliac joint
L. sacrum

Anterior view

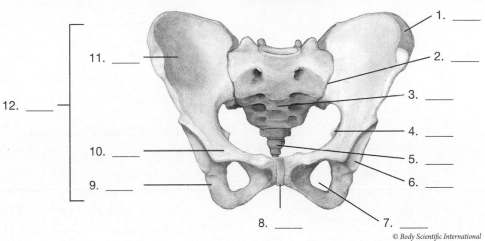

1. ____
2. ____
3. ____
4. ____
5. ____
6. ____
7. ____
8. ____
9. ____
10. ____
11. ____
12. ____

© Body Scientific International

Section 5.4 Vocabulary Review

Match each vocabulary word with its definition.

A. amphiarthrosis
B. articular fibrocartilage
C. ball-and-socket joint
D. bursae
E. condylar joint
F. diarthrosis
G. gliding joint
H. hinge joint
I. ligament
J. pivot joint
K. saddle joint
L. symphysis
M. synarthrosis
N. synchondrosis
O. syndesmosis
P. synovial joint
Q. tendon
R. tendon sheath

____ 1. synovial joint
____ 2. connects bone to bone
____ 3. type of joint at the hip
____ 4. hyaline cartilage that separates the two pubis bones
____ 5. type of joint at the knee
____ 6. connects muscle to bone
____ 7. joint that allows only slight movement
____ 8. meniscus
____ 9. type of joint between the atlas and axis

____ 10. synovial structures surrounding tendons
____ 11. diarthrodial joint
____ 12. type of joint at the base of the thumb
____ 13. capsule filled with synovial fluid
____ 14. type of fibrous joint that allows for little or no movement
____ 15. joint in which one surface is a convex oval and the other is a concave oval
____ 16. diarthrotic joint that allows only sliding motions
____ 17. hyaline cartilage that holds articulating bones together
____ 18. fibrous tissue that binds bones together allowing extremely limited movement

Section 5.4 Study Questions

1. Name and describe the two categories of synarthroses.
2. What are the three categories of joints based on the amount of movement allowed?
3. Describe a gliding joint and give an example of this joint in the body.
4. How many axes of movement are possible in a pivot joint?
5. What types of movements are allowed by a condylar joint?
6. Describe a ball-and-socket joint and give an example of this joint in the body.
7. What is a bursa?
8. What is the function of a tendon sheath?
9. What is a meniscus?
10. What is the difference between tendons and ligaments?

Section 5.4 Labeling
The Knee
Identify the structures in the knee.

Labeling Terms
A. articular capsule
B. articular cartilage
C. fat pad
D. junction of membrane with cartilage
E. lateral meniscus
F. medial meniscus
G. patella
H. synovial membrane

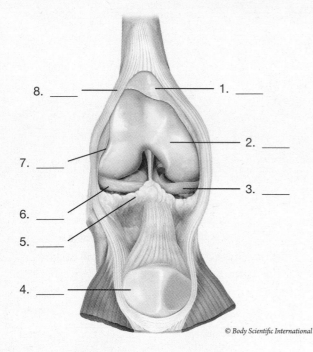

8. ____ ____   1. ____

7. ____

6. ____

5. ____

4. ____

2. ____

3. ____

© Body Scientific International

Section 5.5 Vocabulary Review
Match each vocabulary word with its definition.

A. amenorrhea
B. anorexia nervosa
C. apophysis
D. arthritis
E. bulimia nervosa
F. bursitis
G. dislocation
H. female athlete triad
I. fracture
J. osteoarthritis
K. osteopenia
L. osteoporosis
M. rheumatoid arthritis
N. sprain

____ 1. describes a bone that is not in its socket
____ 2. inflammation of a joint
____ 3. decrease in bone density without a fracture
____ 4. autoimmune disease resulting in destruction of joint tissues

____ 5. inflammation of small capsules in a synovial joint
____ 6. results from overstretching a ligament or tendon
____ 7. absence of a menstrual cycle
____ 8. decrease in bone density characterized by fractures
____ 9. condition that is characterized by eating binges, vomiting, and misuse of laxatives
____ 10. destruction of the articular cartilage in a joint
____ 11. location where a tendon attaches to a bone
____ 12. bone breakage
____ 13. abnormal fear of gaining weight with a distorted view of body image
____ 14. combination of poor eating, amenorrhea, and osteoporosis in women

Section 5.5 Study Questions

1. List and describe seven types of bone fractures.
2. What challenges are researchers encountering in the field of bone tissue engineering?
3. What could result from an injury to an epiphyseal plate?
4. Differentiate between osteopenia and osteoporosis.
5. How do type I osteoporosis and type II osteoporosis differ?
6. What is the female athlete triad?
7. How can osteoporosis be prevented?
8. What is a sprain?
9. What is bursitis?
10. How do osteoarthritis and rheumatoid arthritis differ?

Section 5.5 Labeling
Types of Fractures
Identify each type of fracture

Labeling Terms
A. comminuted fracture
B. crush fracture
C. greenstick fracture
D. impacted fracture
E. spiral fracture
F. stress fracture
G. wedge fracture

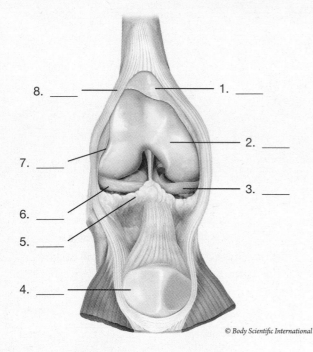
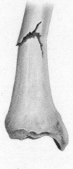
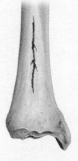

1. ____   2. ____

© Body Scientific International

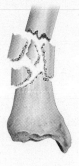 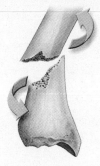

3. _____   4. _____

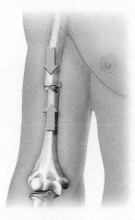 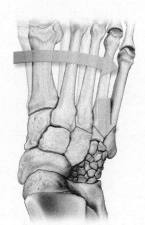

5. _____   6. _____

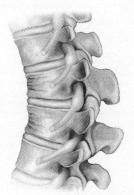

7. _____

© Body Scientific International

Medical Terminology

For each item, identify the word parts and their meanings, and then provide the meaning of the medical term. Use a medical dictionary or the textbook if you need help.

1. dysmenorrhea

   prefix: _____

   meaning: _____

   root/combining form: _____

   meaning: _____

   suffix: _____

   meaning: _____

   meaning of word: _____

2. corticospinal

   root/combining form: _____

   meaning: _____

   root/combining form: _____

   meaning: _____

   suffix: _____

   meaning: _____

   meaning of word: _____

3. hematology

   root/combining form: _____

   meaning: _____

   suffix: _____

   meaning: _____

   meaning of word: _____

4. hemangioma

   root/combining form: _____

   meaning: _____

   root/combining form: _____

   meaning: _____

   suffix: _____

   meaning: _____

   meaning of word: _____

5. arthroscope

    root/combining form: _____

    meaning: _____

    suffix: _____

    meaning: _____

    meaning of word: _____

6. arthralgia

    root/combining form: _____

    meaning: _____

    suffix: _____

    meaning: _____

    meaning of word: _____

7. avascular

    prefix: _____

    meaning: _____

    root/combining form: _____

    meaning: _____

    suffix: _____

    meaning: _____

    meaning of word: _____

8. metaphysis

    prefix: _____

    meaning: _____

    suffix: _____

    meaning: _____

    meaning of word: _____

9. osteochondroma

    root/combining form: _____

    meaning: _____

    root/combining form: _____

    meaning: _____

    suffix: _____

    meaning: _____

    meaning of word: _____

10. osteogenesis

    root/combining form: _____

    meaning: _____

    suffix: _____

    meaning: _____

    meaning of word: _____

Name: _____ Date: _____

Section 6.1 Vocabulary Review

Match each vocabulary word with its definition.

A. agonist
B. antagonist
C. aponeurosis
D. concentric contraction
E. contractility
F. eccentric contraction
G. elasticity
H. endomysium
I. epimysium
J. extensibility
K. fascicle
L. irritability
M. isometric contraction
N. muscle fiber
O. perimysium
P. sarcolemma

_____ 1. sheetlike tendon
_____ 2. connective tissue covering around the entire skeletal muscle
_____ 3. the ability to shorten
_____ 4. muscle contraction with no movement
_____ 5. a muscle cell
_____ 6. contraction that lengthens a muscle
_____ 7. plasma membrane of muscle cell
_____ 8. the skeletal muscle that causes the movement
_____ 9. ability to recoup shape after stretching
_____ 10. the skeletal muscle that stops a movement
_____ 11. contraction that shortens a muscle
_____ 12. bundle of muscle fibers
_____ 13. the ability to be stretched
_____ 14. connective tissue covering around the fascicle
_____ 15. ability to respond to a stimulus
_____ 16. connective tissue covering around each muscle cell

Section 6.1 Study Questions

1. Describe the appearance of the three types of muscle.
2. Explain what parts of a muscle are surrounded by endomysium, perimysium, and epimysium.

3. How do concentric and eccentric contractions differ?
4. If you flex your arm, which roles do the biceps and triceps play?
5. Define the term *irritability* in reference to muscles.
6. What is the function of intercalated discs?
7. How do isometric contractions differ from other types of muscle contractions?
8. What is meant by a tensile force?
9. Which of the three types of muscle are involuntary?
10. How do extensibility and contractility differ?

Section 6.1 Labeling
Organization of Skeletal Muscle

Identify the parts of a muscle and its surrounding structures.

Labeling Terms

A. blood vessel
B. bone
C. endomysium
D. epimysium
E. fascia
F. fascicle
G. muscle fiber
H. perimysium
I. tendon

1. _____
2. _____
3. _____
4. _____
5. _____
6. _____
7. _____
8. _____
9. _____

© Body Scientific International

Name: _____   Date: _____

Section 6.2 Vocabulary Review I

Match each vocabulary word with its definition.

A. acetylcholine
B. action potential
C. all-or-none rule
D. axon
E. axon terminal
F. cross bridges
G. fast-twitch
H. insertion
I. motor neuron
J. motor unit
K. neuromuscular junction
L. origin
M. parallel fiber architecture
N. pennate fiber architecture
O. sarcomere
P. slow-twitch
Q. synaptic cleft
R. tetanus

_____ 1. muscle type that reacts slowly and fatigues slowly

_____ 2. a neurotransmitter

_____ 3. movable attachment site

_____ 4. contractile unit of a muscle

_____ 5. the stalk-like extension off the neuron's cell body

_____ 6. muscle fiber arrangement where fibers all go lengthwise

_____ 7. myosin heads grab onto binding sites on actin

_____ 8. sustained muscle contraction

_____ 9. part of the nervous system that stimulates skeletal muscle

_____ 10. charge when stimulation of a nerve or muscle occurs

_____ 11. motor neuron and all of the muscle fibers it stimulates

_____ 12. immovable attachment site

_____ 13. muscle type that contracts quickly and fatigues quickly

_____ 14. fibers in a motor unit always develop maximum tension when stimulated

_____ 15. muscle fiber arrangement where muscle fibers go diagonally off a tendon

_____ 16. gap between neuron and muscle

_____ 17. part of neuron that connects to individual muscle fibers

_____ 18. link between axon terminal and muscle

Section 6.2 Vocabulary Review II

Match each vocabulary word with its definition.

A. abduction
B. adduction
C. circumduction
D. dorsiflexion
E. eversion
F. extension
G. flexion
H. hyperextension
I. inversion
J. lateral rotation
K. medial rotation
L. opposition
M. plantar flexion
N. pronation
O. supination

_____ 1. pointing the toes

_____ 2. move the sole of the foot outward

_____ 3. lateral movement away from the body

_____ 4. rotation in a circle

_____ 5. decreases the angle between two bones

_____ 6. outward movement in a transverse plane

_____ 7. moving the palm downward

_____ 8. medial movement toward the body

_____ 9. increasing the angle beyond the anatomical position

_____ 10. act of touching any fingers to thumb

_____ 11. inward movement in a transverse plane

_____ 12. movement of the foot up toward the leg

_____ 13. increasing the angle between two bones

_____ 14. lateral rotation with the palm up

_____ 15. sole of foot moves inward

Section 6.2 Study Questions

1. What is the role of acetylcholine in a muscle contraction?

2. What is a sarcomere?

3. If you should decide to run marathons, would you prefer to have more fast-twitch or slow-twitch fibers?

4. How do unipennate, bipennate, and multipennate fiber arrangements differ?

5. What is the formula for mechanical power?

6. How are the origin and insertion of a muscle different?

7. What is sarcopenia?

8. Which movements take place within the sagittal plane?

9. Which movements occur within the frontal plane?

10. Which movements occur within the transverse plane?

Section 6.2 Labeling
Neuromuscular Junction

Identify the parts of the neuromuscular junction.

Labeling Terms

A. acetylcholine receptor sites
B. axon
C. axon terminal

D. diffusing acetylcholine
E. muscle fiber
F. sarcolemma

G. synaptic cleft
H. vesicles containing acetylcholine

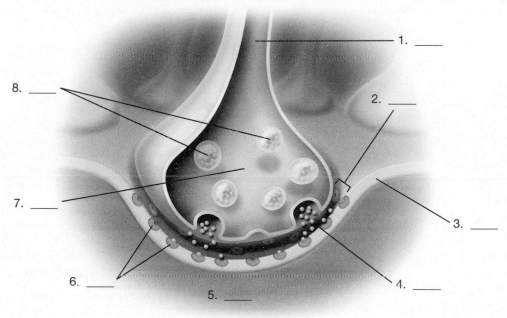

8. ____
7. ____
6. ____
5. ____
1. ____
2. ____
3. ____
4. ____

© *Body Scientific International*

Muscle Fiber Arrangements

Identify the types of muscle fiber arrangements.

Labeling Terms

A. bundled
B. bipennate
C. fusiform
D. multipennate
E. parallel fiber arrangements
F. pennate fiber arrangements
G. triangular
H. unipennate

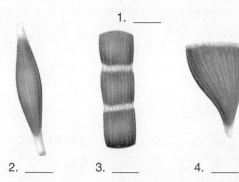

1. ____

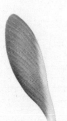

2. ____

3. ____

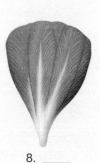

4. ____

5. ____

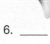

6. ____

7. ____

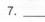

8. ____

© *Body Scientific International*

Directional Movement Terminology

Identify the term for each directional movement.

Labeling Terms

A. abduction	E. eversion	I. inversion	M. pronation
B. adduction	F. extension	J. lateral rotation	N. radial deviation
C. circumduction	G. flexion	K. medial rotation	O. supination
D. dorsiflexion	H. hyperextension	L. plantar flexion	P. ulnar deviation

Sagittal plane movements

1. _____

2. _____

3. _____   4. _____   5. _____

Frontal plane movements

6. _____   7. _____

8. _____   9. _____   10. _____   11. _____

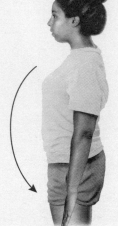
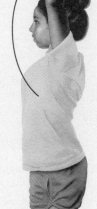
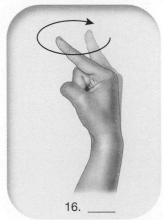
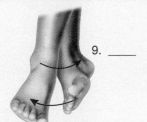
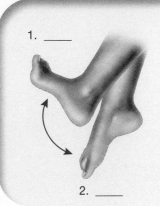
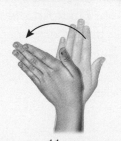
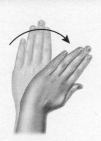
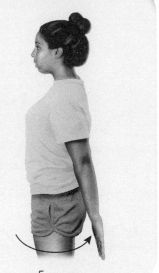
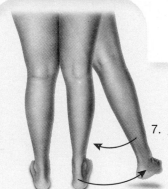

Transverse plane movements

12. _____   13. _____

14. _____   15. _____

Multi-plane movement

16. _____

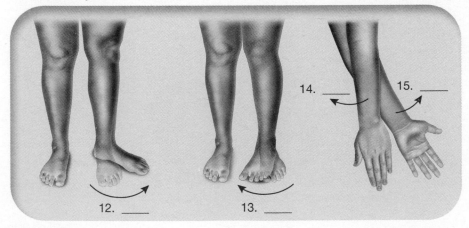

© Body Scientific International

Section 6.3 Vocabulary Review

Match each vocabulary word with its definition.

A. agonist-antagonist pairs
B. diaphragm
C. linea alba
D. rectus sheath
E. rotator cuff

_____ 1. important muscle used for breathing; subdivides ventral body cavity

_____ 2. four muscles at the shoulder joint

_____ 3. muscles that oppose each other

_____ 4. connective tissue around the rectus abdominis muscle

_____ 5. connective tissue that separates rectus abdominis muscle

Section 6.3 Study Questions

1. Which two muscles of the head have a circular orientation?
2. Which muscles of the head and neck are named for the location of nearby bones?
3. If you developed a "double chin," which muscle would most likely be involved in the surgery to correct it?
4. Which muscle allows you to smile and which is involved in a frown?
5. Which abdominal muscle could give you "six-pack abs"?
6. Name the muscles that make up the rotator cuff.
7. Which muscles are named for their size?
8. Name as many muscles as you can that are better seen from a posterior view.
9. Name the four quadriceps muscles.
10. Which three muscles are classified as the hamstrings?

Section 6.3 Labeling

Major Muscles of the Head and Neck

Identify the major muscles of the head and neck.

Labeling Terms

A. buccinator
B. epicranial aponeurosis
C. frontalis

D. masseter
E. nasalis
F. occipitalis

G. orbicularis oculi
H. orbicularis oris
I. platysma

J. sternocleidomastoid
K. temporalis
L. zygomaticus

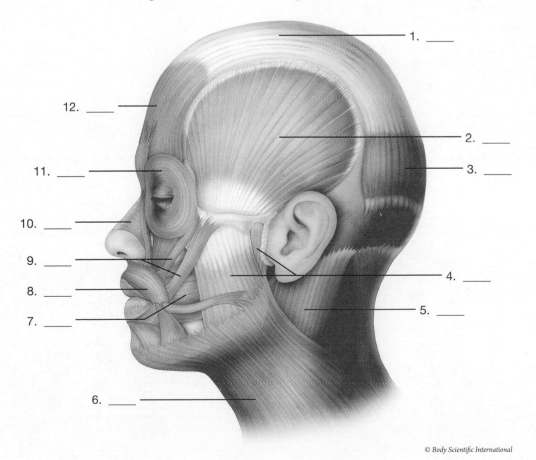

1. _____
2. _____
3. _____
4. _____
5. _____
6. _____
7. _____
8. _____
9. _____
10. _____
11. _____
12. _____

© Body Scientific International

Anterior View of the Trunk

Identify the major muscles in the trunk.

Labeling Terms

A. abdominal aponeurosis
B. external intercostal
C. external oblique
D. external oblique
(cut and pulled back)
E. internal intercostal
F. internal oblique
G. rectus abdominis

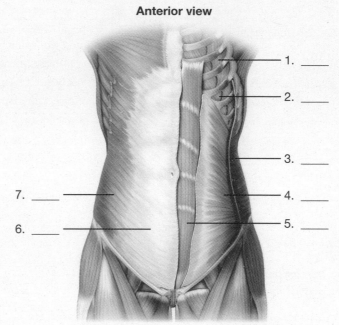

Anterior view

1. ____
2. ____
3. ____
4. ____
5. ____
6. ____
7. ____

© Body Scientific International

Muscles of the Upper Limb

Identify the major muscles and bones of the upper limb.

Labeling Terms

A. biceps brachii
B. brachialis
C. brachioradialis
D. clavicle

E. deltoid
F. humerus
G. lateral head

H. latissimus dorsi
I. long head
J. pectoralis major

K. scapula
L. sternum
M. triceps brachii

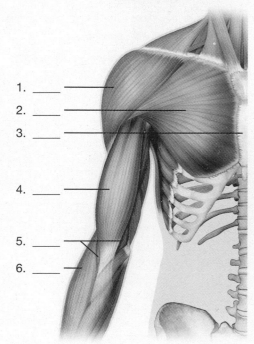

Anterior view

1. ____
2. ____
3. ____
4. ____
5. ____
6. ____

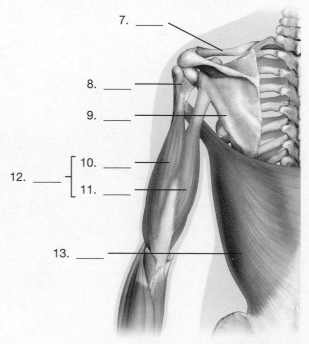

Posterior view

7. ____
8. ____
9. ____
10. ____
11. ____
12. ____
13. ____

© Body Scientific International

Muscles of the Rotator Cuff

Identify the muscles of the rotator cuff.

Labeling Terms

A. acromion
B. clavicle
C. coracoid process
D. glenoid fossa
E. inferior angle
F. infraspinatus
G. rotator cuff
   (SITS) muscles
H. subscapularis
I. supraspinatus
J. teres minor

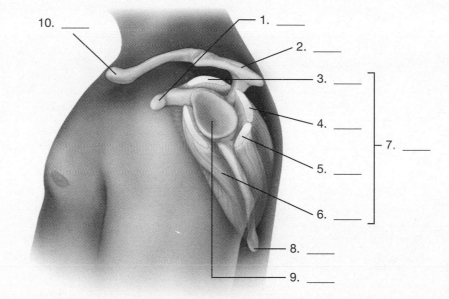

10. ____   1. ____
            2. ____
            3. ____
            4. ____   7. ____
            5. ____
            6. ____
            8. ____
            9. ____

© Body Scientific International

Section 6.4 Vocabulary Review

Match each vocabulary word with its definition.

A. contusion
B. delayed-onset muscle soreness (DOMS)
C. hernia
D. muscle cramps
E. muscle strain
F. muscular dystrophy (MD)
G. myositis ossificans
H. shin splints
I. tendinitis
J. tendinosis

_____ 1. tissue protruding through a muscle
_____ 2. formation of calcium mass in a muscle
_____ 3. inflammation of a tendon
_____ 4. painful spasms in a muscle
_____ 5. bleeding or bruising of a muscle
_____ 6. progressive disorder in which muscle
         is destroyed
_____ 7. pain focused along the tibia
_____ 8. overstretching of a muscle
_____ 9. pain resulting from small muscle tears after
         vigorous exercise
_____ 10. degeneration of a tendon

Section 6.4 Study Questions

1. Describe the three classifications of strains.
2. Explain how a contusion can escalate into myositis ossificans.
3. What are some potential causes of cramps?
4. What are some common causes of low back pain?
5. Explain what is meant by *delayed-onset muscle soreness*.
6. What is the difference between tendinitis and tendinosis?
7. What is swimmer's shoulder?
8. How do tennis elbow and Little Leaguer's elbow differ?
9. What typically causes shin splints?
10. Why is a hernia sometimes a dangerous condition?

Medical Terminology

For each item, identify the word parts and their meanings, and then provide the meaning of the medical term. Use a medical dictionary or the textbook if you need help.

1. bradycardia

   prefix: _____

   meaning: _____

   root/combining form: _____

   meaning: _____

   suffix: _____

   meaning: _____

   meaning of word: _____

2. myometrium

    root/combining form: _____

    meaning: _____

    root/combining form: _____

    meaning: _____

    suffix: _____

    meaning: _____

    meaning of word: _____

3. bradykinesia

    prefix: _____

    meaning: _____

    root/combining form: _____

    meaning: _____

    suffix: _____

    meaning: _____

    meaning of word: _____

4. pericardial

    prefix: _____

    meaning: _____

    root/combining form: _____

    meaning: _____

    suffix: _____

    meaning: _____

    meaning of word: _____

5. myoglobin

    root/combining form: _____

    meaning: _____

    suffix: _____

    meaning: _____

    meaning of word: _____

6. perimetrium

    prefix: _____

    meaning: _____

    root/combining form: _____

    meaning: _____

    suffix: _____

    meaning: _____

    meaning of word: _____

7. periodontal

    prefix: _____

    meaning: _____

    root/combining form: _____

    meaning: _____

    suffix: _____

    meaning: _____

    meaning of word: _____

8. spermatogenesis

    root/combining form: _____

    meaning: _____

    suffix: _____

    meaning: _____

    meaning of word: _____

9. oogenesis

    root/combining form: _____

    meaning: _____

    suffix: _____

    meaning: _____

    meaning of word: _____

10. leiomyosarcoma

    root/combining form: _____

    meaning: _____

    root/combining form: _____

    meaning: _____

    suffix: _____

    meaning: _____

    meaning of word: _____

NOTES

7 The Nervous System

Name: _____ Date: _____

Section 7.1 Vocabulary Review

Match each vocabulary word with its definition.

A. afferent nerves
B. autonomic nervous system
C. axon
D. cell body
E. central nervous system (CNS)
F. dendrites
G. efferent nerves
H. myelin sheath
I. neurilemma
J. neuroglia
K. neuron
L. nodes of Ranvier
M. peripheral nervous system (PNS)
N. somatic nervous system
O. synapse
P. synaptic cleft

_____ 1. brain and spinal cord

_____ 2. gap between neurons

_____ 3. carry impulses toward the brain

_____ 4. areas on an axon with no myelin sheath

_____ 5. all parts of the nervous system except the brain and spinal cord

_____ 6. conducts nerve impulses away from the cell body

_____ 7. junction between a neuron and a muscle, gland, or receptor

_____ 8. part of a neuron that houses the nucleus

_____ 9. division of the nervous system that involves involuntary actions

_____ 10. carry impulses away from the brain

_____ 11. covering of a nerve fiber

_____ 12. division of the nervous system that involves voluntary actions

_____ 13. specialized cell that stimulates muscles or glands

_____ 14. examples include Schwann cells and astrocytes

_____ 15. collect information and send it to the cell body

_____ 16. surrounds the axon of some neurons

Section 7.1 Study Questions

1. How do the central nervous system and peripheral nervous system differ?

2. Neurons can be classified according to function or structure. What are the major categories in each type of classification?

3. What are the major components of a neuron?

4. What are the two subdivisions within the efferent nerves, and what is the function of each?

5. What is an interneuron?

6. What is the difference between Schwann cells and oligodendrocytes?

7. Describe the structure of unipolar, bipolar, and multipolar neurons.

8. What are the functions of microglia and ependymal cells?

9. What is another name for a sensory neuron? For a motor neuron?

10. Distinguish between afferent and efferent nerves.

Section 7.1 Labeling
Parts of a Neuron
Identify the parts of a typical neuron.

Labeling Terms

A. axon
B. axon terminals
C. cell body
D. dendrites

E. myelin sheath
F. neurilemma
G. nodes of Ranvier

H. nucleus
I. postsynaptic cell body
   of another neuron

J. saltatory conduction
K. Schwann cell
L. Schwann cell nucleus

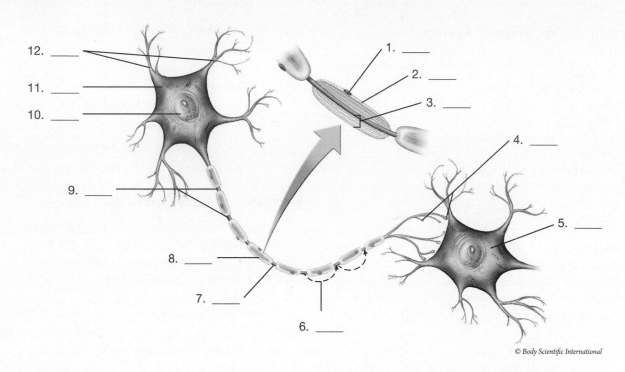

© Body Scientific International

Unipolar Neuron
Identify the parts of a unipolar neuron.

Labeling Terms

A. axon terminals
B. cell body
C. central process of axon

D. dendrites
E. initial segment
F. peripheral process of axon

Unipolar neuron

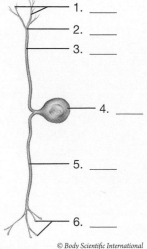

1. ____
2. ____
3. ____
4. ____
5. ____
6. ____

© Body Scientific International

Section 7.2 Vocabulary Review
Match each vocabulary word with its definition.

A. action potential
B. autonomic reflexes
C. conductivity
D. depolarized
E. neurotransmitter
F. polarized

G. reflexes
H. refractory period
I. repolarization
J. saltatory conduction
K. somatic reflexes

____ 1. state in which the inside of a cell membrane is more negatively charged than the outside

____ 2. time between the end of an action potential and repolarization

____ 3. predictable, involuntary response to a stimulus

____ 4. transmission of an action potential in a myelinated axon

____ 5. electrical charge that travels down an axon

____ 6. involuntary stimuli sent to cardiac and smooth muscle when stimulated

____ 7. return to a polarized state after depolarization

____ 8. ability of a neuron to transmit a nerve impulse

_____ 9. state in which the inside of a cell membrane is more positively charged than the outside

_____ 10. involuntary stimuli sent to skeletal muscles when stimulated

_____ 11. chemical released from axon terminals

Section 7.2 Study Questions

1. Explain the concept of conductivity.

2. Define the term *action potential*.

3. Explain the processes of polarization, depolarization, and repolarization in a neuron.

4. Explain what is meant by a refractory period.

5. What factors influence the speed of nerve impulse transmission?

6. Which excitatory neurotransmitter activates muscle fibers?

7. What information can be obtained from microneurography?

8. What is a reflex?

9. Give an example of a somatic reflex.

10. What are the two categories of reflexes, and how do they differ?

Section 7.2 Labeling

Synapse Site

Identify the parts of a synapse site.

Labeling Terms

A. axon
B. axon terminal
C. diffusing neurotransmitter
D. muscle fiber
E. neurotransmitter receptor sites

F. sarcolemma
G. synaptic cleft
H. vesicle containing neurotransmitter

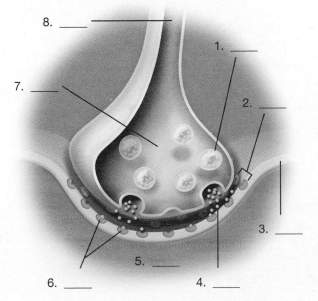

8. _____
1. _____
7. _____
2. _____
3. _____
6. _____
5. _____
4. _____

© Body Scientific International

Section 7.3 Vocabulary Review

Match each vocabulary word with its definition.

A. cerebellum
B. cerebrum
C. diencephalon
D. epithalamus
E. fissures
F. frontal lobes
G. hypothalamus
H. lobes
I. medulla oblongata
J. meninges

K. midbrain
L. occipital lobes
M. parietal lobes
N. pons
O. primary motor cortex
P. primary somatic sensory cortex
Q. spinal cord
R. temporal lobes
S. thalamus

_____ 1. part of the cerebrum responsible for vision

_____ 2. portion of the brain stem that deals with breathing rate

_____ 3. responsible for balance and coordinated muscle movement

_____ 4. part of the central nervous system in addition to the brain

_____ 5. deep grooves in the brain

_____ 6. protective membranes around the brain and spinal cord

_____ 7. largest part of the human brain

_____ 8. part of the cerebrum responsible for speech, memory, and emotion

_____ 9. portion of the frontal lobes that sends messages to the skeleton

_____ 10. area behind the frontal lobes that integrates information from skin and muscles

_____ 11. superior part of the brain stem that serves as a relay station

_____ 12. contains the pineal gland

_____ 13. largest part of the diencephalon; sends sensory information to the cerebral cortex

_____ 14. contains the thalamus, hypothalamus, and epithalamus

_____ 15. divisions of the brain separated by sulci

_____ 16. outer region of the parietal lobes that interprets sensory impulses

_____ 17. region located behind the forehead; involved in advanced thought and speech

_____ 18. part of the diencephalon that controls heart rate and blood pressure

_____ 19. lowest part of the brain stem; controls breathing and heart rates

Section 7.3 Study Questions

1. What are the four basic anatomic regions of the brain?

2. What are the basic functions of the various lobes of the cerebrum?

3. How do the primary motor cortex and the primary somatic sensory cortex differ?

4. Name the three meninges.
5. Name two locations relative to the spinal cord that contain cerebrospinal fluid.
6. What is the location and function of the cerebellum?
7. Which diagnostic tests are useful to study the brain?

8. List the three divisions of the brain stem and describe the functions of each.
9. Explain the function of the blood-brain barrier.
10. What causes some brain tissue to be white and other tissue to be gray?

Section 7.3 Labeling
The Brain

Identify the lobes and features of the brain.

Labeling Terms

A. brain stem
B. central sulcus
C. cerebellum
D. frontal lobe
E. lateral sulcus
F. occipital lobe
G. parietal lobe
H. parieto-occipital sulcus
I. temporal lobe

Lobes of the brain

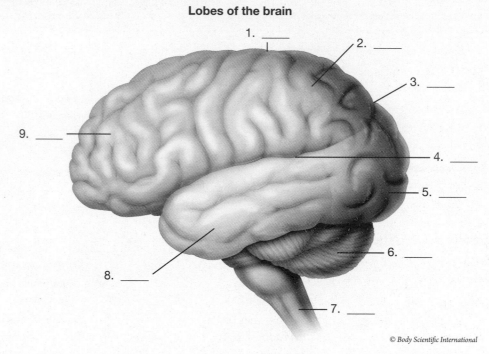

1. ____
2. ____
3. ____
4. ____
5. ____
6. ____
7. ____
8. ____
9. ____

© Body Scientific International

Diencephalon

Identify the structures in and around the diencephalon.

Labeling Terms

A. brain stem
B. diencephalon (thalamus in view)
C. medulla oblongata
D. midbrain
E. pons
F. spinal cord

Anterior view

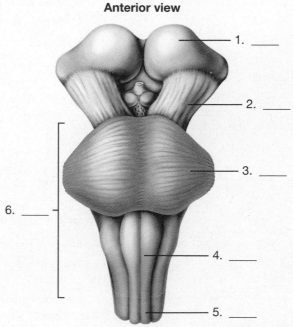

1. ____
2. ____
3. ____
4. ____
5. ____
6. ____

© Body Scientific International

Spinal Cord

Identify the layers and regions of the spinal cord.

Labeling Terms

A. arachnoid mater
B. central canal
C. dorsal (posterior) horn of gray matter
D. dorsal root ganglion

E. dorsal root of spinal nerve
F. dura mater
G. lateral horn of gray matter
H. pia mater

I. spinal nerve
J. ventral (anterior) horn of gray matter
K. ventral root of spinal nerve
L. white matter

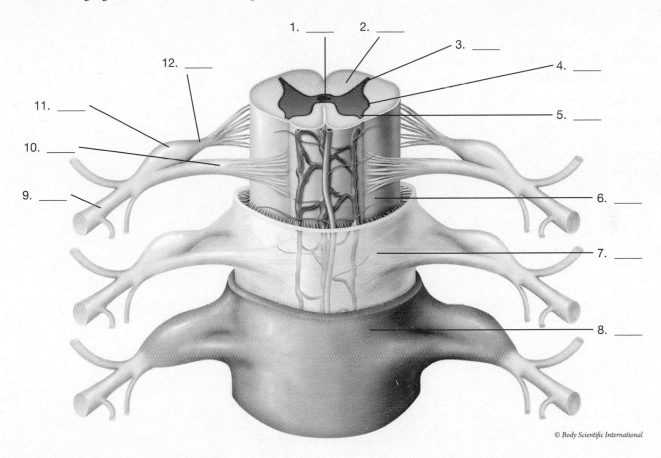

© Body Scientific International

Section 7.4 Vocabulary Review

Match each vocabulary word with its definition.

A. acetylcholine
B. cranial nerves
C. craniosacral division
D. dorsal ramus
E. endoneurium
F. epineurium
G. ganglion
H. norepinephrine

I. paravertebral ganglia
J. perineurium
K. plexuses
L. postganglionic neuron
M. preganglionic neuron
N. spinal nerves
O. thoracolumnar division
P. ventral ramus

_____ 1. twelve pairs of nerves that originate in the brain

_____ 2. thirty-one pairs of nerves off of the spinal cord

_____ 3. connective tissue covering of individual nerve fibers

_____ 4. nerve cell bodies that are parallel to the spinal cord

_____ 5. a neurotransmitter that stimulates skeletal muscle

_____ 6. another name for the parasympathetic system

_____ 7. a neurotransmitter that brings about a fight-or-flight response

_____ 8. second, unmyelinated neuron that transmits impulses from the CNS

_____ 9. another name for the sympathetic division of the ANS

_____ 10. posterior spinal nerves that send motor impulses to posterior trunk muscles

_____ 11. anterior division of spinal nerves that supply areas in anterior and lateral trunk

_____ 12. first, myelinated neuron in a series that transmits impulses from the CNS

_____ 13. complex nerve interconnections

_____ 14. connective tissue covering of a fascicle of nerve fibers

_____ 15. mass of cell bodies that acts as a junction between neurons

_____ 16. connective tissue covering of an entire nerve

Section 7.4 Study Questions

1. What are the three connective tissue coverings of a nerve?

2. How many cranial nerves are present in the human body? How many spinal nerves?

3. What is the cauda equina?

4. Which three cranial nerves control eye movements?

5. Which cranial nerve is the only one to have functions outside of the head and neck?

6. How do the dorsal and ventral rami differ?

7. Name the four spinal nerve plexuses and the areas they supply.

8. Describe the fight-or-flight response.

9. What causes shingles?

10. What is the role of the parasympathetic division of the ANS?

Section 7.4 Labeling
Structure of a Nerve

Identify the structures and features of a typical nerve.

Labeling Terms

A. axon
B. blood vessels
C. endoneurium

D. epineurium
E. fascicle

F. myelin sheath
G. perineurium

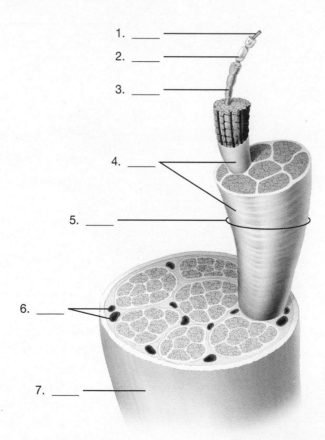

1. ____
2. ____
3. ____
4. ____
5. ____
6. ____
7. ____

© Body Scientific International

Cranial Nerves

Identify each of the twelve cranial nerves.

Labeling Terms

A. abducens
B. accessory
C. facial

D. glossopharyngeal
E. hypoglossal
F. oculomotor

G. olfactory
H. optic
I. trigeminal

J. trochlear
K. vagus
L. vestibulocochlear

CNS Connection

- [ ] Cerebrum
- [ ] Diencephalon
- [ ] Midbrain
- [ ] Pons
- [ ] Medulla oblongata

1. ____   I

2. ____   II

3. ____

III

4. ____   IV

5. ____   VI

6. ____

7. ____

8. ____

9. ____

10. ____   VIII

11. ____   V

12. ____   VII

X

XI

IX

XII

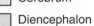
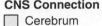
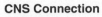
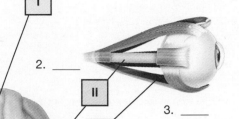
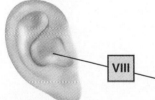
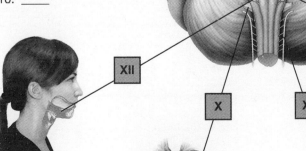
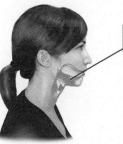

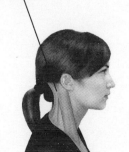

© *Body Scientific International*

Section 7.5 Vocabulary Review

Match each vocabulary word with its definition.

A. Alzheimer's disease (AD)
B. cerebral palsy
C. dementia
D. epilepsy
E. Huntington's disease
F. meningitis
G. multiple sclerosis (MS)
H. paraplegia
I. Parkinson's disease
J. quadriplegia
K. traumatic brain injury

_____ 1. inflammation of membranes around the brain and spinal cord

_____ 2. inability to move the torso or legs

_____ 3. type of progressive dementia

_____ 4. destruction of myelin sheaths

_____ 5. inability to move anything below the neck

_____ 6. loss of function in two or more areas of cognition

_____ 7. genetic disease characterized by inability to control movements and emotions

_____ 8. condition resulting from brain damage before or during birth

_____ 9. disorder in which patients exhibit tremors and muscle weakness

_____ 10. damage resulting from trauma to the head

_____ 11. characterized by seizures

Section 7.5 Study Questions

1. What are the symptoms of a traumatic brain injury?

2. How are sports officials attempting to prevent damage from head injuries associated with contact sports?

3. Which types of spinal cord damage result in quadriplegia and paraplegia?

4. What are the symptoms and treatment options for an individual with meningitis?

5. How is Parkinson's disease treated?

6. What is the cause of Huntington's disease?

7. What signs may indicate that an epilepsy patient may be about to have a seizure?

8. Why is multiple sclerosis classified as an autoimmune disease?

9. List potential causes of cerebral palsy.

10. What is the most common cause of dementia?

Medical Terminology

For each item, identify the word parts and their meanings, and then provide the meaning of the medical term. Use a medical dictionary or the textbook if you need help.

1. myelitis

    root/combining form: _____

    meaning: _____

    suffix: _____

    meaning: _____

    meaning of word: _____

2. cranial

    root/combining form: _____

    meaning: _____

    suffix: _____

    meaning: _____

    meaning of word: _____

3. arachnodactyly

    root/combining form: _____

    meaning: _____

    root/combining form: _____

    meaning: _____

    suffix: _____

    meaning: _____

    meaning of word: _____

4. myelofibrosis

    root/combining form: _____

    meaning: _____

    root/combining form: _____

    meaning: _____

    suffix: _____

    meaning: _____

    meaning of word: _____

5. microcephaly

    prefix: _____

    meaning: _____

    root/combining form: _____

    meaning: _____

    suffix: _____

    meaning: _____

    meaning of word: _____

6. arachnoiditis

    root/combining form: _____

    meaning: _____

    suffix: _____

    meaning: _____

    meaning of word: _____

7. craniotomy

    root/combining form: _____

    meaning: _____

    suffix: _____

    meaning: _____

    meaning of word: _____

8. microembolus

    prefix: _____

    meaning: _____

    root/combining form: _____

    meaning: _____

    suffix: _____

    meaning: _____

    meaning of word: _____

9. myelogram

    root/combining form: _____

    meaning: _____

    suffix: _____

    meaning: _____

    meaning of word: _____

10. microsomia

    prefix: _____

    meaning: _____

    root/combining form: _____

    meaning: _____

    suffix: _____

    meaning: _____

    meaning of word: _____

NOTES

Name: _____   Date: _____

Section 8.1 Vocabulary Review

Match each vocabulary word with its definition.

A. aqueous humor
B. choroid
C. ciliary body
D. ciliary glands
E. cones
F. conjunctiva
G. cornea
H. extrinsic muscles
I. fovea centralis
J. iris
K. lacrimal glands
L. lens
M. optic chiasma
N. optic nerve
O. optic tracts
P. pupil
Q. retina
R. rods
S. sclera
T. suspensory ligaments
U. tarsal glands
V. vitreous humor

_____ 1. secrete oil along eyelids

_____ 2. controls size of pupil

_____ 3. secrete tears

_____ 4. where the two optic nerves cross

_____ 5. muscles attached to the outside of the eye

_____ 6. middle layer of the wall of the eye

_____ 7. part of the eye that contains rods and cones

_____ 8. liquid that maintains intraocular pressure

_____ 9. part of the optic nerve fibers that go beyond the optic chiasma

_____ 10. detect colors

_____ 11. opening in the iris

_____ 12. located between the choroid and the iris

_____ 13. gel-type material in posterior chamber

_____ 14. transparent material at the anterior surface of the eye

_____ 15. white outer layer of the eye

_____ 16. takes visual sensory signals to the occipital lobe of the brain

_____ 17. structures that attach the lens to the ciliary body

_____ 18. point of greatest visual acuity

_____ 19. glands located between the eyelashes

_____ 20. cells activated by dim light

_____ 21. membrane that lines the eyelid

_____ 22. transparent, flexible structure behind the iris

Section 8.1 Study Questions

1. In what ways are the eyes protected by surrounding structures?

2. Describe the three layers of the eye.

3. Compare and contrast aqueous humor and vitreous humor.

4. Describe the functions of the two types of sensory receptor cells in the retina.

5. What is the difference between wet and dry macular degeneration?

6. What is a cataract and how is this condition treated?

7. How do myopia and hyperopia differ?

8. How is amblyopia treated?

9. How is color blindness inherited?

10. What is presbyopia?

Section 8.1 Labeling
Extrinsic Muscles of the Eye

Identify the extrinsic muscles that control the eye.

Labeling Terms

A. inferior oblique muscle
B. inferior rectus muscle
C. lateral rectus muscle
D. medial rectus muscle
E. superior oblique muscle
F. superior rectus muscle

1. _____
2. _____
3. _____
4. _____
5. _____
6. _____

© Body Scientific International

Internal Structures of the Eye

Identify the internal structures of the eye.

Labeling Terms

A. aqueous humor (liquid filling)
B. choroid layer
C. ciliary body

D. conjunctiva
E. cornea
F. iris
G. lens

H. optic nerve
I. pupil
J. retina
K. sclera

L. sphincter pupillae
M. suspensory ligaments
N. vitreous humor (liquid filling)

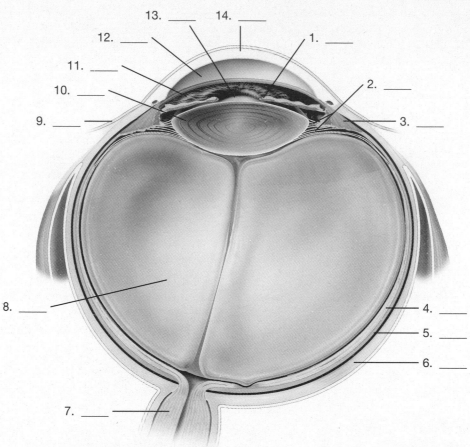

13. ____   14. ____
12. ____
11. ____
10. ____
9. ____
8. ____
7. ____

1. ____
2. ____
3. ____
4. ____
5. ____
6. ____

© Body Scientific International

Section 8.2 Vocabulary Review

Match each vocabulary word with its definition.

A. auditory canal
B. auricle
C. bony labyrinth
D. ceruminous glands
E. cochlea
F. cochlear duct
G. endolymph
H. Eustachian tube
I. incus
J. malleus

K. membranous labyrinth
L. organ of Corti
M. ossicles
N. oval window
O. perilymph
P. semicircular canals
Q. stapes
R. tympanic membrane
S. vestibule
T. vestibulocochlear nerve

____ 1. secrete earwax in the auditory canal
____ 2. collective name for the hammer, anvil, and stirrup
____ 3. equalizes pressure on both sides of the eardrum
____ 4. cranial nerve that relates to hearing and equilibrium
____ 5. fluid in the bony labyrinth

____ 6. membranous structures within the bony labyrinth
____ 7. outer ear
____ 8. hammer
____ 9. opening that connects middle ear to the inner ear
____ 10. snail-shaped inner ear area
____ 11. contains hearing receptors in a cochlear duct
____ 12. fluid in the membranous labyrinth
____ 13. stirrup
____ 14. winding tunnel in the inner ear
____ 15. eardrum
____ 16. area in inner ear that contains semicircular canals
____ 17. anvil
____ 18. membranous labyrinth within the cochlea
____ 19. connects the outer ear to the eardrum
____ 20. three loops in the inner ear

Section 8.2 Study Questions

1. What is the purpose of cerumen?
2. What bony structures are located in the middle ear, and what is their function?
3. What is the function of the Eustachian tube?
4. Describe the process involved in hearing.
5. How is equilibrium maintained in the body?
6. What is amusia?
7. How does a cochlear implant differ from a standard hearing aid?
8. What is tinnitus?
9. What is the difference between otitis externa, otitis media, and otitis interna?
10. What is Ménière's disease?

Section 8.2 Labeling
Anatomy of the Ear
Identify the structures of the ear.

Labeling Terms

A. anvil (incus)
B. auditory canal (external acoustic meatus)
C. auricle
D. cochlea
E. Eustachian tube
F. external (outer) ear
G. hammer (malleus)
H. internal (inner) ear
I. middle ear (tympanic cavity)
J. ossicles
K. oval window
L. round window
M. semicircular canals
N. stirrup (stapes)
O. tympanic membrane (eardrum)
P. vestibule
Q. vestibulocochlear nerve

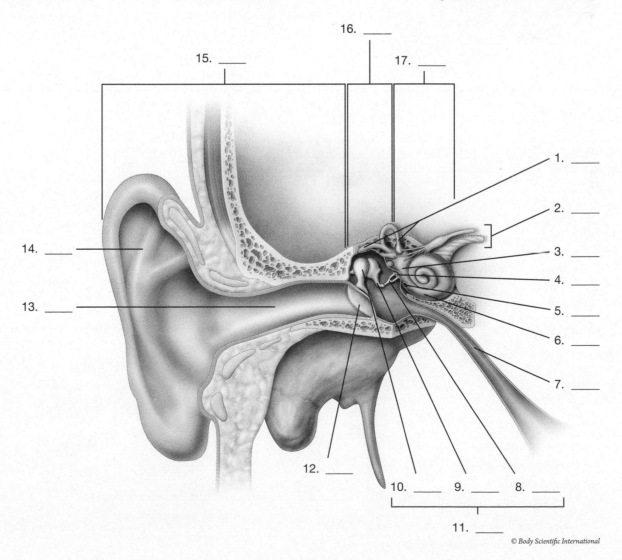

16. ____
15. ____
17. ____
1. ____
2. ____
14. ____
3. ____
4. ____
13. ____
5. ____
6. ____
7. ____
12. ____
10. ____   9. ____   8. ____
11. ____

© Body Scientific International

Structures of the Inner Ear

Identify the structures of the inner ear.

Labeling Terms

A. bony labyrinth (contains perilymph)
B. cochlea
C. cochlear nerve
D. membranous labyrinth (contains endolymph)
E. oval window
F. semicircular canals
G. vestibular nerve
H. vestibule

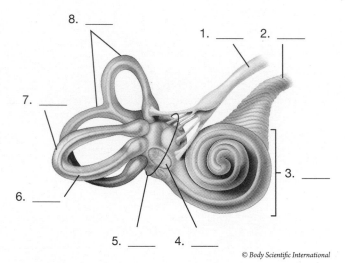

8. _____
1. _____   2. _____
7. _____
6. _____
3. _____
5. _____   4. _____

© Body Scientific International

Section 8.3 Vocabulary Review

Match each vocabulary word with its definition.

A. antihistamines
B. gustatory cells
C. gustatory hairs
D. histamines
E. limbic system
F. olfactory bulb
G. olfactory hairs
H. olfactory nerve
I. olfactory receptor cells
J. olfactory region
K. papillae
L. septum
M. tastants
N. taste buds
O. taste pores

_____ 1. filaments in taste buds

_____ 2. openings in the tops of taste buds

_____ 3. emotional brain

_____ 4. compounds that stimulate gustatory hairs

_____ 5. medications that oppose the activities of histamines

_____ 6. filaments that extend from olfactory cells

_____ 7. area in the nasal cavity where olfactory cells are located

_____ 8. sensory receptors for taste

_____ 9. thickened area of the olfactory nerve

_____ 10. bumps on the tongue that contain taste buds

_____ 11. sensors responsible for smell

_____ 12. cranial nerve that transports information to the brain to identify odors

_____ 13. sensory receptors inside the taste buds

_____ 14. molecules that produce nasal congestion and drainage

_____ 15. wall between the two sides of the nose

Section 8.3 Study Questions

1. Why is it difficult to detect an odor when you have a head cold?

2. Describe the events that occur in the olfactory region.

3. How are the sense of smell and the limbic system related?

4. Describe the relationship between histamines and antihistamines.

5. What advantages do dogs have in regard to their olfactory sensation?

6. Where are the taste buds located?

7. Describe the structure of a taste bud.

8. Which three cranial nerves transport taste sensations to the brain?

9. What are the five basic taste categories?

10. When people decide if they like the taste of something, what other factors are taken into consideration in addition to information from taste buds?

Section 8.3 Labeling

Taste Bud

Identify the parts of a typical taste bud.

Labeling Terms

A. afferent nerves
B. gustatory (taste) cells
C. gustatory hairs
D. papilla on surface of tongue
E. taste pore
F. tongue

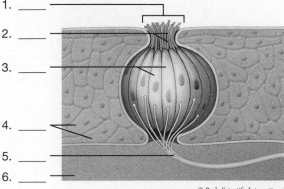

1. _____
2. _____
3. _____
4. _____
5. _____
6. _____

© Body Scientific International

Medical Terminology

For each item, identify the word parts and their meanings, and then provide the meaning of the medical term. Use a medical dictionary or the textbook if you need help.

1. presbyatrics

    root/combining form: _____

    meaning: _____

    root/combining form: _____

    meaning: _____

    suffix: _____

    meaning: _____

    meaning of word: _____

2. amblyopia

    root/combining form: _____

    meaning: _____

    suffix: _____

    meaning: _____

    meaning of word: _____

3. aquaphobia

    root/combining form: _____

    meaning: _____

    suffix: _____

    meaning: _____

    meaning of word: _____

4. aural

    root/combining form: _____

    meaning: _____

    suffix: _____

    meaning: _____

    meaning of word: _____

5. ophthalmopathy

    root/combining form: _____

    meaning: _____

    suffix: _____

    meaning: _____

    meaning of word: _____

6. aquagenic

    root/combining form: _____

    meaning: _____

    suffix: _____

    meaning: _____

    meaning of word: _____

7. auricular

    root/combining form: _____

    meaning: _____

    suffix: _____

    meaning: _____

    meaning of word: _____

8. ophthalmitis

    root/combining form: _____

    meaning: _____

    suffix: _____

    meaning: _____

    meaning of word: _____

9. lacrimation

    root/combining form: _____

    meaning: _____

    suffix: _____

    meaning: _____

    meaning of word: _____

10. vasculitis

　　root/combining form: _____

　　meaning: _____

　　suffix: _____

　　meaning: _____

　　meaning of word: _____

9 The Endocrine System

Name: _____   Date: _____

Section 9.1 Vocabulary Review

Match each vocabulary word with its definition.

A. amino acid-derived hormones
B. cyclic adenosine monophosphate (cAMP)
C. downregulated
D. epinephrine
E. glucagon
F. hormonal control
G. hormones
H. humoral control
I. hypothalamic non-releasing hormones
J. hypothalamic releasing hormones
K. insulin
L. neural control
M. steroid hormones
N. upregulated

_____   1. decreased
_____   2. release of hormones to control other endocrine glands
_____   3. water-soluble hormones made of proteins
_____   4. stimulation of endocrine glands by nerve fibers
_____   5. hormone made by the pancreas to lower the glucose level
_____   6. secreted to cause the fight-or-flight mechanism
_____   7. powerful chemical messengers
_____   8. a second messenger derived from ATP
_____   9. hormone made by the pancreas to raise the blood sugar
_____   10. increased
_____   11. produced by the hypothalamus to inhibit the release of pituitary hormones
_____   12. lipid-based hormones
_____   13. produced by the hypothalamus to stimulate the release of pituitary hormones
_____   14. hormone release based on monitoring content of body fluids

Section 9.1 Study Questions

1. What is the difference between endocrine glands and exocrine glands?

2. What are hormones, and what type of activities do they control?

3. How are hormones transported through the body?
4. How do steroid hormones produce an effect within a target cell?
5. How do amino acid-derived hormones produce an effect within a target cell?
6. Describe neural control of hormone secretion.
7. Describe hormonal control of hormone secretion.
8. What is humoral control?
9. How do hormones help maintain homeostasis?
10. How does the hypothalamus control body temperature?

Section 9.1 Labeling
The Endocrine System

Identify glands and organs of the endocrine system.

Labeling Terms

A. adrenal glands
B. hypothalamus
C. ovary (female)
D. pancreas
E. parathyroid gland
F. pineal gland
G. pituitary gland
H. testis (male)
I. thyroid gland
J. thymus gland

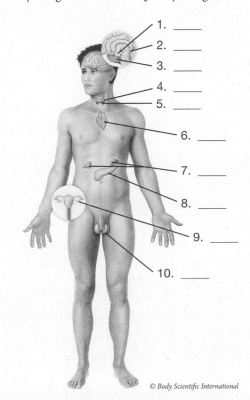

1. _____
2. _____
3. _____
4. _____
5. _____
6. _____
7. _____
8. _____
9. _____
10. _____

© Body Scientific International

Section 9.2 Vocabulary Review

Match each vocabulary term with its definition.

A. adrenal cortex
B. adrenal glands
C. adrenal medulla
D. anterior pituitary
E. ovaries
F. pancreas
G. parathyroid glands
H. pineal gland
I. pituitary gland
J. posterior pituitary
K. scrotum
L. testes
M. thymus
N. thyroid gland
O. tropic hormones

_____ 1. secretes insulin and glucagon

_____ 2. sac containing the testes

_____ 3. contains two lobes: one secretes six hormones and the other stores two made by the hypothalamus

_____ 4. produces T_3, T_4, and calcitonin

_____ 5. secretes estrogen and progesterone

_____ 6. glands that sit on top of the kidneys

_____ 7. four glands that are located behind the thyroid

_____ 8. produce testosterone

_____ 9. outer layer of the gland that sits on top of the kidneys

_____ 10. lobe that secretes six hormones

_____ 11. hormones that act on other glands

_____ 12. inner layer of the gland that sits on top of the kidneys

_____ 13. secretes thymosin

_____ 14. secretes melatonin

_____ 15. stores two hormones made by the hypothalamus

Section 9.2 Study Questions

1. How does the hypothalamus control the pituitary gland?

2. What two hormones are made by the hypothalamus?

3. What are the four tropic hormones released by the pituitary gland?

4. Compare the functions of the two lobes of the pituitary gland.

5. Which hormones are released by the thyroid gland?

6. Describe the relationship between parathyroid hormone and calcitonin.

7. What hormones are produced by the medulla and cortex of the adrenal glands?

8. How does the pancreas work to control blood sugar?

9. What is the function of thymosin?

10. Explain the role of the pineal gland.

Section 9.2 Labeling
The Posterior Pituitary

Identify the hormones released by the posterior pituitary gland and the glands and tissues affected.

Labeling Terms

A. ADH
B. anterior pituitary
C. axon terminals
D. hypothalamic neuroendocrine input
E. hypothalamus
F. infundibulum
G. kidneys
H. mammary glands
I. oxytocin
J. posterior pituitary
K. uterine muscles

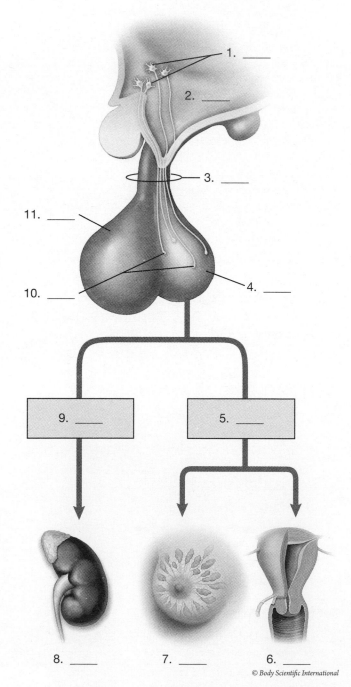

© Body Scientific International

The Adrenal Glands

Identify the layers and structures of the adrenal gland.

Labeling Terms

A. adrenal cortex
B. adrenal medulla
C. cortex

D. glucocorticoid-secreting area
E. kidney
F. medulla

G. mineralocorticoid-secreting area
H. sex hormone-secreting area

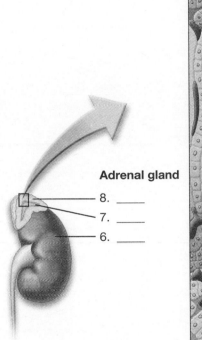

Adrenal gland

8. _____
7. _____
6. _____

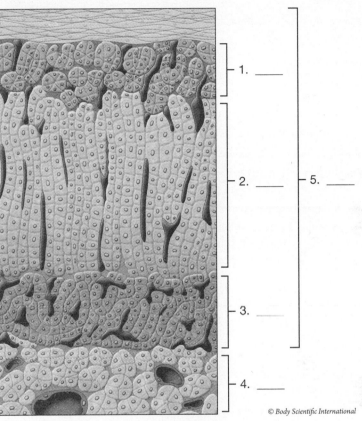

1. _____
2. _____   5. _____
3. _____
4. _____

© Body Scientific International

Section 9.3 Vocabulary Review

Match each vocabulary term with its definition.

A. acromegaly
B. Addison's disease
C. Cushing's syndrome
D. diabetes insipidus
E. diabetes mellitus
F. dwarfism
G. goiter
H. Graves' disease
I. hypercalcemia
J. hyperglycemia

K. hyperthyroidism
L. hypothyroidism
M. insulin resistance
N. myxedema
O. neonatal hypothyroidism
P. peripheral neuropathy
Q. tetany
R. thyroiditis
S. type I diabetes mellitus
T. type II diabetes mellitus

_____ 1. hyposecretion of antidiuretic hormone

_____ 2. hyposecretion of human growth hormone

_____ 3. severe hyposecretion of T_3 and T_4

_____ 4. severe hypersecretion of T_3 and T_4

_____ 5. hypersecretion of human growth hormone after the growing years

_____ 6. destruction of cells producing insulin

_____ 7. inflammation of the thyroid

_____ 8. hypersecretion of hormones from the adrenal cortex

_____ 9. high glucose levels

_____ 10. high calcium levels

_____ 11. enlarged thyroid gland

_____ 12. peripheral nerve damage due to diabetes mellitus

_____ 13. hyposecretion of hormones from the adrenal cortex

_____ 14. involves downregulation of insulin receptors

_____ 15. muscles in a constant state of contraction

_____ 16. insufficient T_3 and T_4 in infants

_____ 17. condition present in type II diabetes

_____ 18. underactive thyroid gland

_____ 19. overactive thyroid gland

_____ 20. inability to regulate glucose levels

Section 9.3 Study Questions

1. What conditions can result from inappropriate levels of human growth hormone?
2. In what way are diabetes insipidus and diabetes mellitus similar? How are they different?
3. What are the symptoms of hyperthyroidism and hypothyroidism?
4. Why is hypothyroidism particularly damaging to infants?
5. What are the symptoms of the two parathyroid disorders?
6. What condition can result from a disorder of the adrenal medulla?
7. Describe the disorders that involve hyposecretion and hypersecretion of hormones from the adrenal cortex.
8. Which blood tests can help diagnose diabetes?
9. How do type I and type II diabetes differ?
10. What ill effects can result from uncontrolled diabetes?

Medical Terminology

For each item, identify the word parts and their meanings, and then provide the meaning of the medical term. Use a medical dictionary or the textbook if you need help.

1. ectothermic

    prefix: _____

    meaning: _____

    root/combining form: _____

    meaning: _____

    suffix: _____

    meaning: _____

    meaning of word: _____

2. thermophobia

    root/combining form: _____

    meaning: _____

    suffix: _____

    meaning: _____

    meaning of word: _____

3. hypercarbia

    prefix: _____

    meaning: _____

    root/combining form: _____

    meaning: _____

    suffix: _____

    meaning: _____

    meaning of word: _____

4. hypoallergenic

    prefix: _____

    meaning: _____

    root/combining form: _____

    meaning: _____

    suffix: _____

    meaning: _____

    meaning of word: _____

5. exogenous

    prefix: _____

    meaning: _____

    root/combining form: _____

    meaning: _____

    suffix: _____

    meaning: _____

    meaning of word: _____

6. exotropia

    prefix: _____

    meaning: _____

    suffix: _____

    meaning: _____

    meaning of word: _____

7. gonadarche

    root/combining form: _____

    meaning: _____

    suffix: _____

    meaning: _____

    meaning of word: _____

8. hyperbaric

    prefix: _____

    meaning: _____

    root/combining form: _____

    meaning: _____

    suffix: _____

    meaning: _____

    meaning of word: _____

9. hyperbilirubinemia

    prefix: _____

    meaning: _____

    root/combining form: _____

    meaning: _____

    suffix: _____

    meaning: _____

    meaning of word: _____

10. endothermic

    prefix: _____

    meaning: _____

    root/combining form: _____

    meaning: _____

    suffix: _____

    meaning: _____

    meaning of word: _____

NOTES

Name: _____ Date: _____

Section 10.1 Vocabulary Review

Match each vocabulary word with its definition.

A. alveoli
B. bronchioles
C. cardiopulmonary system
D. ciliated epithelium
E. epiglottis
F. larynx
G. mediastinum
H. nares
I. nasal conchae
J. olfactory receptors
K. palate
L. pharynx
M. pleural sac
N. pores of Kohn
O. primary bronchi
P. sinuses
Q. surfactant
R. thyroid cartilage
S. tonsils
T. trachea

____ 1. air-filled cavities within the skull
____ 2. prevents alveoli from collapsing
____ 3. where gas exchange occurs
____ 4. separates oral and nasal cavities
____ 5. involve the sense of smell
____ 6. tube inferior to the larynx
____ 7. throat
____ 8. flap that covers respiratory pathways while swallowing
____ 9. voice box
____ 10. includes lungs, heart, and blood vessels
____ 11. nostrils
____ 12. branches extending from the trachea
____ 13. area between the lungs
____ 14. lymphatic tissue in the pharynx
____ 15. allows for travel between alveoli
____ 16. ductwork between tertiary bronchi and alveoli
____ 17. Adam's apple
____ 18. tissue lining with hair-like projections
____ 19. three bones that create nasal pathways
____ 20. encloses the lungs

Section 10.1 Study Questions

1. What are the functions of the upper respiratory tract?
2. How is the air filtered as it passes through the nose?
3. What are the functions of the sinuses?
4. What are the three divisions of the pharynx?
5. What is the function of the epiglottis?
6. What are the functions of the C-shaped rings in the trachea?
7. Which structures in the lungs contain cartilaginous rings?
8. How does surfactant aid the lungs?
9. How many lobes are in each lung?
10. Describe the pleura surrounding the lungs.

Section 10.1 Labeling
Upper Respiratory System
Identify the structures of the upper respiratory system.

Labeling Terms

A. epiglottis	F. lingual tonsil	I. nasal vestibular region	N. thyroid cartilage
B. esophagus	G. naris	J. palatine tonsil	O. tongue
C. frontal sinus	H. nasal conchae	K. pharyngeal tonsil	P. trachea
D. hard palate	(superior, middle,	L. soft palate	Q. uvula
E. laryngopharynx	and inferior)	M. sphenoid sinus	R. vocal fold

The upper respiratory tract

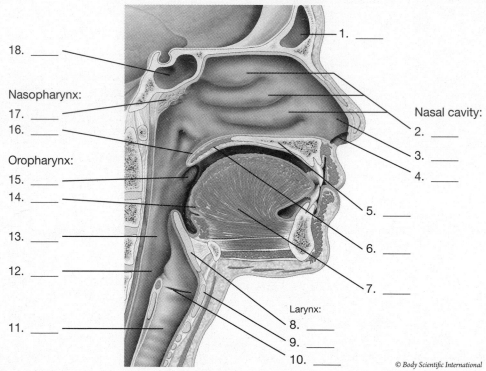

18. ____

Nasopharynx:
17. ____
16. ____

Oropharynx:
15. ____
14. ____

13. ____

12. ____

11. ____

1. ____

Nasal cavity:
2. ____
3. ____
4. ____

5. ____

6. ____

7. ____

Larynx:
8. ____
9. ____
10. ____

© Body Scientific International

Lower Respiratory Tract
Identify the structures of the lower respiratory tract.

Labeling Terms

A. alveoli
B. bronchiole
C. cartilaginous rings
D. larynx
E. primary bronchi
F. secondary bronchi
G. tertiary bronchi
H. trachea

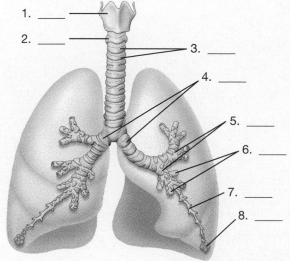

1. ____
2. ____
3. ____
4. ____
5. ____
6. ____
7. ____
8. ____

© Body Scientific International

Section 10.2 Vocabulary Review

Match each vocabulary word with its definition.

A. alveolar capillary membrane
B. chemoreceptors
C. expiration
D. expiratory reserve volume (ERV)
E. external respiration
F. forced expiratory volume in one second (FEV$_1$)
G. forced expiratory volume in one second/forced vital capacity (FEV$_1$/FVC)
H. functional residual capacity (FRC)
I. Hering-Breuer reflex
J. inspiration
K. inspiratory reserve volume (IRV)
L. internal respiration
M. mechanoreceptors
N. partial pressure
O. pulmonary ventilation
P. residual volume (RV)
Q. respiration
R. respiratory gas transport
S. tidal volume (TV)
T. total lung capacity (TLC)
U. vital capacity (VC)

_____ 1. gas exchange

_____ 2. amount of air that normally passes in and out while breathing

_____ 3. structure through which gases pass during gas exchange in the alveoli

_____ 4. amount of air that can be expired in one second

_____ 5. amount of air that must remain in lungs to keep them inflated

_____ 6. cells that respond to chemical stimuli

_____ 7. air flowing into the lungs

_____ 8. additional amount of air that can be exhaled after normal exhalation

_____ 9. process by which oxygen and carbon dioxide travel to and from the lungs and tissues

_____ 10. ratio that shows the expiratory power of the lungs

_____ 11. prevents overinflation of the lungs

_____ 12. total amount of air that can be forced out of the lungs after maximum inspiration

_____ 13. mechanics of moving air in and out of lungs

_____ 14. air flowing out of the lungs

_____ 15. gas exchange between capillaries and tissues of the body

_____ 16. the pressure of a gas when it is mixed with other gases

_____ 17. gas exchange between capillaries and alveoli in the lungs

_____ 18. vital capacity + residual volume

_____ 19. ERV+ RV

_____ 20. additional amount of air that can be inhaled after a normal inhalation

_____ 21. type of sensory cells that involve respiration

Section 10.2 Study Questions

1. What is the difference between internal respiration and external respiration?
2. Explain how Boyle's law applies to breathing.
3. Define Fick's Law of Diffusion.
4. How is oxygen transported in the bloodstream?
5. How is carbon dioxide transported in the bloodstream?
6. List four examples of nonrespiratory air maneuvers.
7. How do neural factors help to control respiration?
8. How do central and peripheral chemoreceptors differ?
9. Describe the various volume measurements used to assess lung capacity.
10. Which conditions can be identified based on a patient's FEV$_1$ and FEV$_1$/FVC values?

Section 10.2 Labeling

Lung Tissue

Identify the components of lung tissue.

Labeling Terms

A. alveolar basement membrane
B. alveolar sac
C. alveolar wall
D. capillary basement membrane
E. capillary wall
F. cluster of alveoli
G. red blood cell
H. red blood cell in capillary

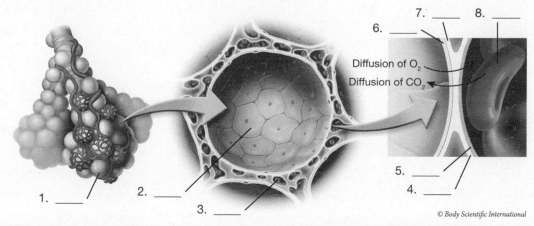

Diffusion of O$_2$
Diffusion of CO$_2$

1. _____   2. _____   3. _____   4. _____   5. _____   6. _____   7. _____   8. _____

© Body Scientific International

Lung Volume

Identify the results from a static lung volume spirometer test.

Labeling Terms

A. expiratory reserve volume (ERV) 1200 mL
B. inspiratory reserve volume (IRV) 3100 mL
C. residual volume (RV) 1200 mL
D. tidal volume (TV) 500 mL
E. total lung capacity (TLC) 6000 mL
F. vital capacity (VC) 4800 mL

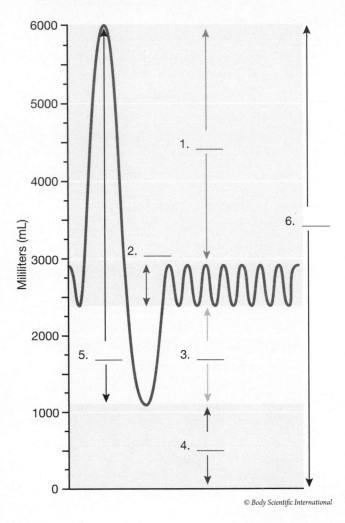

© Body Scientific International

Section 10.3 Vocabulary Review

Match each vocabulary word with its definition.

A. acute bronchitis
B. asthma
C. bronchospasms
D. chronic bronchitis
E. chronic obstructive pulmonary disease (COPD)
F. emphysema
G. hyperventilation
H. influenza
I. laryngitis
J. nasal pharyngitis
K. pharyngitis
L. pneumonia
M. sinusitis
N. tonsillitis
O. tuberculosis (TB)

_____ 1. inflammation of the voice box

_____ 2. long-term inflammation of the bronchi and production of excess mucus

_____ 3. common viral infection that targets the respiratory system

_____ 4. temporary inflammation of the bronchi and production of excess mucus

_____ 5. disease involving bronchospasms

_____ 6. inflammation of the throat

_____ 7. contagious bacterial infection of the lungs

_____ 8. infection of the lungs, commonly from bacteria or a virus

_____ 9. inflammation of the lymphatic structures of the respiratory system

_____ 10. inflammation of the air-filled cavities in the skull

_____ 11. contractions that occur during an asthma attack

_____ 12. category that includes emphysema and chronic bronchitis

_____ 13. inflammation of the nose and throat

_____ 14. type of COPD characterized by chronic inflammation of the lungs

_____ 15. rapid breathing rate to compensate for poor gas exchange

Section 10.3 Study Questions

1. List four common upper respiratory illnesses.
2. What are the symptoms of influenza?
3. List four things you can do to protect yourself and prevent the spread of upper respiratory infections.
4. What is acute bronchitis?
5. How is pneumonia diagnosed?
6. What is tuberculosis?
7. What is chronic obstructive pulmonary disease (COPD)? List two common examples.
8. How are emphysema and chronic bronchitis different?
9. What is asthma?
10. What are the risk factors for developing lung cancer?

Medical Terminology

For each item, identify the word parts and their meanings, and then provide the meaning of the medical term. Use a medical dictionary or the textbook if you need help.

1. bronchoscopy

   root/combining form: _____

   meaning: _____

   suffix: _____

   meaning: _____

   meaning of word: _____

2. pneumocyte

   root/combining form: _____

   meaning: _____

   suffix: _____

   meaning: _____

   meaning of word: _____

3. bronchopulmonary

   root/combining form: _____

   meaning: _____

   root/combining form: _____

   meaning: _____

   suffix: _____

   meaning: _____

   meaning of word: _____

4. rhinorrhea

   root/combining form: _____

   meaning: _____

   suffix: _____

   meaning: _____

   meaning of word: _____

5. pneumatic

   root/combining form: _____

   meaning: _____

   suffix: _____

   meaning: _____

   meaning of word: _____

6. bronchiectasis

   root/combining form: _____

   meaning: _____

   suffix: _____

   meaning: _____

   meaning of word: _____

7. pneumothorax

   root/combining form: _____

   meaning: _____

   root/combining form: _____

   meaning: _____

   meaning of word: _____

8. rhinotomy

   root/combining form: _____

   meaning: _____

   suffix: _____

   meaning: _____

   meaning of word: _____

9. nasolacrimal

    root/combining form: _____

    meaning: _____

    root/combining form: _____

    meaning: _____

    suffix: _____

    meaning: _____

    meaning of word: _____

10. bronchiolitis

    root/combining form: _____

    meaning: _____

    suffix: _____

    meaning: _____

    meaning of word: _____

11 The Blood

Name: _____ Date: _____

Section 11.1 Vocabulary Review

Match each vocabulary word with its definition.

A. buffy coat
B. coagulation
C. diapedesis
D. endothelial cells
E. erythrocytes
F. erythropoiesis
G. erythropoietin (EPO)
H. fibrin
I. fibrinolysis
J. formed elements
K. hematocrit
L. hematopoietic cells
M. hemoglobin
N. hemolysis
O. hemostasis
P. hypoxia
Q. leukocytes
R. mesenchymal cells
S. phagocytosis
T. plasma
U. platelet plug
V. platelets
W. prothrombin
X. prothrombin activator (PTA)
Y. red blood cells (RBCs)
Z. thrombocytes
AA. white blood cells (WBCs)

_____ 1. hormone that encourages bone marrow to make more RBCs

_____ 2. RBCs, WBCs, and platelets

_____ 3. process of making RBCs

_____ 4. platelets

_____ 5. filament made by the combination of thrombin and fibrinogen

_____ 6. layer between the RBCs and plasma in a centrifuged specimen

_____ 7. below-normal oxygen

_____ 8. type of formed element that fights infections

_____ 9. process by which WBCs engulf and digest a foreign object

_____ 10. process of clot formation to stop bleeding

_____ 11. protein in blood that forms thrombin

_____ 12. type of formed elements that carry oxygen

_____ 13. mass formed by a cluster of platelets

_____ 14. process in which thrombin and fibrinogen form fibrin

_____ 15. red blood cells

_____ 16. liquid portion of blood

_____ 17. cells that develop into tissues of the circulatory and lymphatic systems

_____ 18. percentage of blood that consists of RBCs

_____ 19. type of formed elements that form clots

_____ 20. molecule in RBCs that carries oxygen

_____ 21. lining of all blood vessels

_____ 22. break down fibrin to dissolve a clot

_____ 23. precursor to blood cells

_____ 24. rupture of RBCs

_____ 25. process in which blood passes from a blood vessel into the tissues

_____ 26. protein that activates fibrinogen

_____ 27. technical name for WBCs

Section 11.1 Study Questions

1. What are the functions of blood?
2. Describe the composition of blood.
3. List the proteins found in plasma.
4. Describe the appearance of erythrocytes.
5. What is the function of erythropoietin?
6. What is phagocytosis?
7. Explain the process of diapedesis.
8. Distinguish among the five basic types of leukocytes.
9. What are thrombocytes?
10. Describe the steps that occur in hemostasis.

Section 11.1 Labeling
Composition of Blood
Identify the components of blood.

Labeling Terms
A. blood vessel
B. plasma
C. platelets
D. red blood cells
E. white blood cells

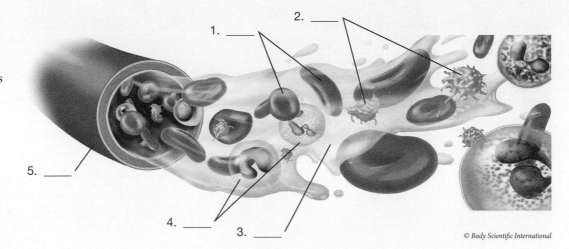

© Body Scientific International

Formed Elements
Identify the formed elements of blood.

Labeling Terms
A. basophil
B. eosinophil
C. lymphocyte
D. monocyte
E. neutrophil
F. platelets
G. red bone marrow
H. red blood cells
I. white blood cells
J. yellow bone marrow

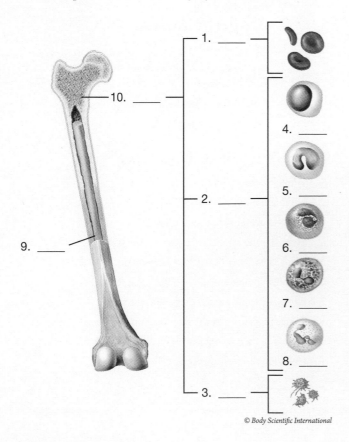

© Body Scientific International

Section 11.2 Vocabulary Review
Match each vocabulary word with its definition.

A. agglutination   E. Rh factor
B. antibodies   F. RhoGAM
C. antigens   G. universal donor
D. erythroblastosis fetalis   H. universal recipient

_____ 1. the clumping of cells

_____ 2. serum given to Rh-negative women to prevent the formation of anti-Rh$^+$ antibodies

_____ 3. type O blood

_____ 4. proteins on the surface of an RBC surface that help distinguish between self and non-self

_____ 5. type AB blood

_____ 6. proteins that react to specific antigens

_____ 7. example of an antigen that is present on the surface of RBCs

_____ 8. condition caused by maternal antibodies crossing the placenta to attack the baby's RBCs

Section 11.2 Study Questions

1. What are the four main blood types?

2. What is an antigen?

3. What is the function of an antibody?

4. Which blood type is considered the universal recipient? Which is the universal donor?

5. What would occur if a patient were given an incompatible blood transfusion?

6. Describe the antigens and antibodies that are present in each of the four blood types.

7. Name all of the blood types that each of the four types could safely receive.

8. What is the Rh factor?

9. What is erythroblastosis fetalis?

10. How does RhoGAM prevent the formation of the anti-Rh⁺ antibody?

Section 11.3 Vocabulary Review

Match each vocabulary word with its definition.

A. acute lymphocytic leukemia (ALL)
B. acute myeloid leukemia (AML)
C. anemia
D. aplastic anemia
E. chelation therapy
F. chronic lymphocytic leukemia (CLL)
G. chronic myeloid leukemia (CML)
H. complete blood count (CBC)
I. embolus
J. hemophilia
K. iron deficient anemia
L. jaundice
M. leukemia
N. multiple myeloma
O. pernicious anemia
P. phlebotomy
Q. polycythemia
R. sickle cell anemia
S. thalassemia
T. thrombus

_____ 1. clot traveling in the bloodstream

_____ 2. removing excess iron from the blood

_____ 3. overproduction of lymphocytes; most common leukemia in children

_____ 4. lack of a clotting factor

_____ 5. clot within an intact vein

_____ 6. diagnostic test that determines the number of RBCs, WBCs, and platelets in the blood

_____ 7. abnormally low number of RBCs

_____ 8. low level of iron due to insufficient hemoglobin/RBCs

_____ 9. drawing blood

_____ 10. disease with abnormally-shaped RBCs

_____ 11. general term for blood cancer that causes overproduction of abnormal WBCs

_____ 12. condition in which there are too many RBCs

_____ 13. overproduction of myeloblasts; most common leukemia in adults

_____ 14. results in a yellowish skin color

_____ 15. leukemia often seen in middle-aged adults, involving overproduction of lymphocytes

_____ 16. disease in which the body has difficulty producing normal hemoglobin and RBCs

_____ 17. cancer affecting the plasma cells in the bone marrow

_____ 18. leukemia with overproduction of granulocytes

_____ 19. condition in which the bone marrow stem cells have trouble making new RBCs

_____ 20. reduced intestinal absorption of vitamin B₁₂, which is necessary for RBC production

Section 11.3 Study Questions

1. What information can be obtained from a complete blood count (CBC)?

2. What is anemia?

3. How can you distinguish among iron-deficient anemia, aplastic anemia, and pernicious anemia?

4. What is sickle cell anemia?

5. What is another name for thalassemia?

6. What are the potential causes of jaundice?

7. Describe the disease hemophilia.

8. What is polycythemia?

9. List and describe the four types of leukemia.

10. What is multiple myeloma?

Medical Terminology

For each item, identify the word parts and their meanings, and then provide the meaning of the medical term. Use a medical dictionary or the textbook if you need help.

1. erythroleukemia

   root/combining form: _____

   meaning: _____

   root/combining form: _____

   meaning: _____

   suffix: _____

   meaning: _____

   meaning of word: _____

2. hypoglycemia

   prefix: _____

   meaning: _____

   root/combining form: _____

   meaning: _____

   suffix: _____

   meaning: _____

   meaning of word: _____

3. leukodystrophy

    root/combining form: _____

    meaning: _____

    prefix: _____

    meaning: _____

    suffix: _____

    meaning: _____

    meaning of word: _____

4. mononucleosis

    prefix: _____

    meaning: _____

    root/combining form: _____

    meaning: _____

    suffix: _____

    meaning: _____

    meaning of word: _____

5. erythema

    root/combining form: _____

    meaning: _____

    suffix: _____

    meaning: _____

    meaning of word: _____

6. leukoplakia

    root/combining form: _____

    meaning: _____

    suffix: _____

    meaning: _____

    meaning of word: _____

7. hyperleukocytosis

    prefix: _____

    meaning: _____

    root/combining form: _____

    meaning: _____

    root/combining form: _____

    meaning: _____

    suffix: _____

    meaning: _____

    meaning of word: _____

8. erythrophobia

    root/combining form: _____

    meaning: _____

    suffix: _____

    meaning: _____

    meaning of word: _____

9. leukemoid

    root/combining form: _____

    meaning: _____

    suffix: _____

    meaning: _____

    meaning of word: _____

10. erythromelalgia

    root/combining form: _____

    meaning: _____

    root/combining form: _____

    meaning: _____

    suffix: _____

    meaning: _____

    meaning of word: _____

12 The Cardiovascular System

Name: _____   Date: _____

Section 12.1 Vocabulary Review

Match each vocabulary word with its definition.

A. aorta
B. aortic valve
C. atrioventricular (AV) valves
D. cardiac output
E. cardiomyocytes
F. diastole
G. endocardium
H. epicardium
I. fibrous pericardium
J. inferior vena cava
K. interatrial septum
L. interventricular septum
M. mediastinum
N. mitral valve
O. myocardium
P. papillary muscle
Q. parietal pericardium
R. pulmonary valve
S. semilunar valves
T. serous pericardium
U. stroke volume
V. superior vena cava
W. systole
X. tricuspid valve
Y. vasoconstriction
Z. vasodilation

_____ 1. area between the lungs
_____ 2. inner lining of the heart
_____ 3. valve between the right ventricle and the lungs
_____ 4. time of least pressure in the heart
_____ 5. largest artery in the body
_____ 6. heart muscle layer
_____ 7. increase in blood vessel diameter
_____ 8. wall between the two upper chambers
_____ 9. collects deoxygenated blood from areas above the heart

_____ 10. cardiac muscle cells
_____ 11. amount of blood that is pumped out of the heart in one minute
_____ 12. strong outer wall of the pericardium
_____ 13. valve between the left atrium and left ventricle
_____ 14. wall between the two lower chambers
_____ 15. outermost layer of the heart
_____ 16. layer of the pericardium between the fibrous layer and the pericardial cavity
_____ 17. time of most pressure in the heart
_____ 18. attached to chordae tendineae in the ventricles
_____ 19. valve between the left ventricle and the aorta
_____ 20. includes aortic and pulmonary valves
_____ 21. includes tricuspid and mitral valves
_____ 22. decrease in blood vessel diameter
_____ 23. collects deoxygenated blood from areas below the heart
_____ 24. volume of blood pumped per beat
_____ 25. valve between the right atrium and right ventricle
_____ 26. part of the pericardium that consists of parietal and visceral layers

Section 12.1 Study Questions

1. Describe the location of the heart.
2. Where are the four valves in the heart located?
3. How does the function of the atrioventricular and semilunar valves differ?
4. Describe the structure of the pericardium.
5. Describe the layers of the heart.
6. Which half of the heart contains deoxygenated blood? Which has oxygenated blood?
7. What is diastole?
8. What events are represented by systole?
9. How is mean arterial pressure calculated?
10. What is the formula for cardiac output?

Section 12.1 Labeling
Layers of the Pericardium
Identify the layers of the pericardium.

Labeling Terms
A. endocardium
B. epicardium
   (serous pericardium)
C. fibrous pericardium
D. left atrium
E. myocardium
F. parietal pericardium
G. pericardial cavity
H. pericardium
I. pulmonary trunk

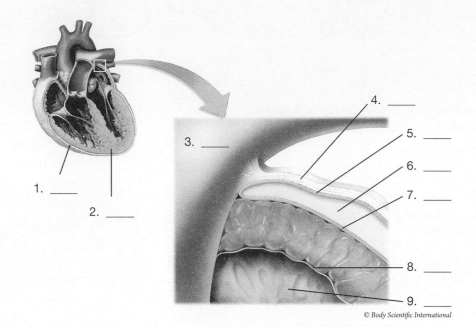

1. ____
2. ____
3. ____
4. ____
5. ____
6. ____
7. ____
8. ____
9. ____

© Body Scientific International

Chambers, Valves, and Vessels of the Heart
Identify the structures of the heart.

Labeling Terms
A. aortic arch
B. aortic valve
C. bicuspid (mitral) valve
D. chordae tendineae
E. descending aorta
F. inferior vena cava
G. interventricular septum
H. left atrium
I. left pulmonary artery
   to left lung
J. left pulmonary veins
K. left ventricle
L. myocardium
M. papillary muscles
N. pulmonary trunk
O. pulmonary valve
P. right atrium
Q. right pulmonary artery
   to right lung
R. right pulmonary veins
S. right ventricle
T. superior vena cava
U. tricuspid valve

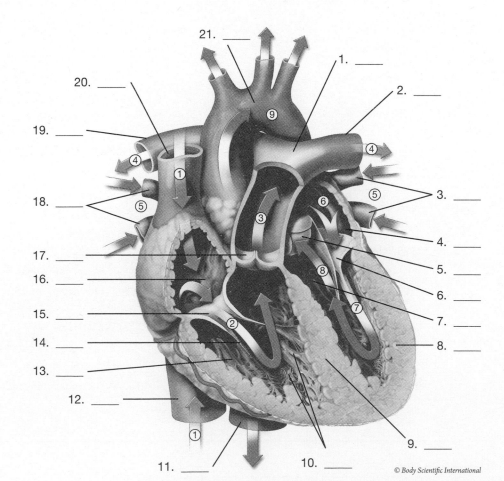

21. ____
20. ____
19. ____
18. ____
17. ____
16. ____
15. ____
14. ____
13. ____
12. ____
11. ____
10. ____

1. ____
2. ____
3. ____
4. ____
5. ____
6. ____
7. ____
8. ____
9. ____

© Body Scientific International

Name: _____   Date: _____

Section 12.2 Vocabulary Review

Match each vocabulary word with its definition.

A. atrioventricular (AV) node
B. Bachmann's bundle
C. baroreceptors
D. bundle branches
E. bundle of His
F. chemoreceptors
G. depolarize
H. mechanoreceptors
I. Purkinje fibers
J. repolarize
K. sinoatrial (SA) node

_____ 1. transmits impulses throughout the ventricles

_____ 2. takes impulses from the AV node to the Purkinje fibers

_____ 3. pacemaker of the heart

_____ 4. tract between the left and right atria

_____ 5. restore original polarity

_____ 6. located in the atria, aortic arch, and carotid arteries to detect changes in blood pressure

_____ 7. change of resting polarity to cause contraction of the heart muscle

_____ 8. transmits impulses from the SA node to the bundle of His

_____ 9. sense stretching in tissues

_____ 10. transmit impulses from the bundle of His to the Purkinje fibers

_____ 11. located in the aortic arch and carotid bodies

Section 12.2 Study Questions

1. What structure is known as the natural pacemaker of the heart?

2. Where is the cardiac center located?

3. Which external factors influence the cardiac center?

4. How does the sympathetic nervous system affect the heart rate?

5. What effect does the parasympathetic nervous system produce on the heart rate?

6. What are baroreceptors?

7. How do chemoreceptors and mechanoreceptors differ?

8. How would you estimate the maximal heart rate for a patient?

9. How do beta blockers affect a patient's heart rate?

10. What is the pathway of conduction through the heart?

Section 12.2 Labeling
Conduction System of the Heart

Identify elements of the heart's conduction system.

Labeling Terms

A. atrioventricular (AV) node
B. Bachmann's bundle
C. bundle of His
D. internodal pathways
E. left atrium
F. Purkinje fibers
G. right and left bundle branches
H. right atrium
I. sinoatrial (SA) node (pacemaker)

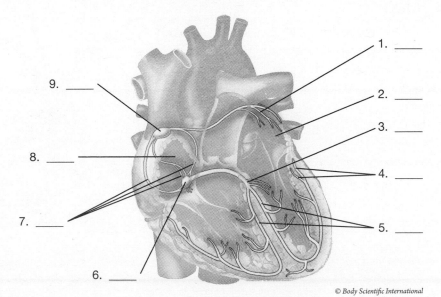

1. _____
2. _____
3. _____
4. _____
5. _____
6. _____
7. _____
8. _____
9. _____

© Body Scientific International

Section 12.3 Vocabulary Review

Match each vocabulary word with its definition.

A. aortic arch
B. arteries
C. arterioles
D. capillaries
E. capillary beds
F. coronary sinus
G. ductus arteriosus
H. foramen ovale
I. hepatic portal system
J. precapillary sphincter
K. pulmonary circulation
L. systemic circulation
M. tunica externa
N. tunica intima
O. tunica media
P. veins
Q. venules

_____ 1. layer of a blood vessel that contains smooth muscle
_____ 2. largest vessels carrying oxygenated blood
_____ 3. collects deoxygenated blood from the heart itself
_____ 4. located between the ascending and descending aorta
_____ 5. part of circulatory system in which blood picks up nutrients from the liver
_____ 6. small vessels carrying deoxygenated blood
_____ 7. network of blood vessels that participate in gas exchange
_____ 8. vessels carrying oxygenated blood between arteries and capillaries
_____ 9. innermost layer of a blood vessel
_____ 10. process that carries oxygen around the body and returns it to the heart
_____ 11. hole between the interatrial wall in a fetus
_____ 12. small blood vessels that participate in gas exchange
_____ 13. outermost layer of a blood vessel
_____ 14. large blood vessels that carry deoxygenated blood back to the heart
_____ 15. connects the left pulmonary artery to the descending aorta in a fetus
_____ 16. smooth muscle that controls blood in the capillaries
_____ 17. process that carries blood to the lungs and back to the heart

Section 12.3 Study Questions

1. Describe the three layers of the wall of a blood vessel.
2. How does the structure of arteries and veins differ?
3. What is the function of a precapillary sphincter?
4. How does the structure of a capillary differ from that of other blood vessels?
5. How do skeletal muscles in the extremities help propel blood back to the heart?
6. Describe pulmonary circulation.
7. How does systemic circulation differ from pulmonary circulation?
8. How is blood supplied to the heart itself?
9. What is the function of the hepatic portal system?
10. Name two structures that are only present in fetal circulation.

Section 12.3 Labeling
Arteries Arising from the Aorta

Identify arteries that arise from the aorta.

Labeling Terms

A. arch of aorta
B. ascending aorta
C. brachiocephalic artery
D. descending aorta
E. left common carotid artery
F. left coronary artery
G. left subclavian artery
H. right common carotid artery
I. right coronary artery
J. right subclavian artery

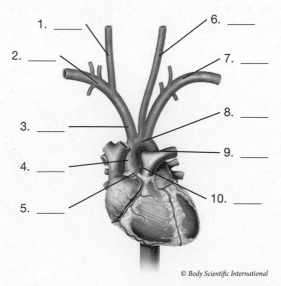

© Body Scientific International

Major Arteries

Identify the major arteries in the human body.

Labeling Terms

A. anterior tibial artery
B. aorta
C. arcuate artery
D. axillary artery
E. brachial artery
F. brachiocephalic artery
G. celiac trunk
H. common iliac artery
I. coronary artery
J. dorsalis pedis artery
K. external carotid artery
L. external iliac artery
M. femoral artery
N. gonadal artery
O. intercostal artery
P. inferior mesenteric artery
Q. internal carotid artery
R. internal iliac artery
S. left common carotid artery
T. lumbar artery
U. popliteal artery
V. posterior tibial artery
W. radial artery
X. renal artery
Y. right common carotid artery
Z. subclavian artery
AA. superior mesenteric artery
BB. ulnar artery
CC. vertebral artery

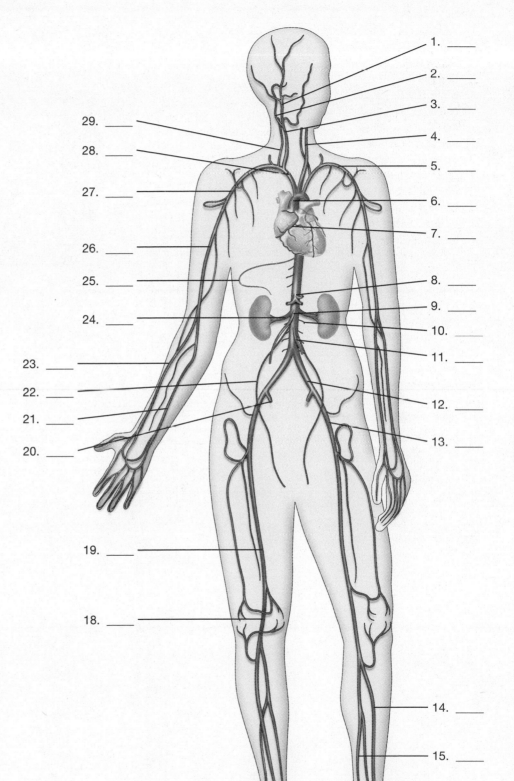

1. ____
2. ____
3. ____
4. ____
5. ____
6. ____
7. ____
8. ____
9. ____
10. ____
11. ____
12. ____
13. ____
14. ____
15. ____
16. ____
17. ____
18. ____
19. ____
20. ____
21. ____
22. ____
23. ____
24. ____
25. ____
26. ____
27. ____
28. ____
29. ____

© Body Scientific International

Major Veins

Identify the major veins in the human body.

Labeling Terms

A. anterior tibial vein
B. axillary vein
C. basilic vein
D. brachial vein
E. cephalic vein
F. common iliac vein
G. dorsal digital veins
H. dorsal venous arch
I. external iliac vein
J. external jugular vein
K. femoral vein
L. gonadal vein
M. great cardiac vein
N. great saphenous vein
O. hepatic vein
P. inferior vena cava
Q. internal iliac vein
R. internal jugular vein
S. left brachiocephalic vein
T. median cubital vein
U. popliteal vein
V. posterior tibial vein
W. radial vein
X. renal vein
Y. right brachiocephalic vein
Z. subclavian vein
AA. superior vena cava
BB. ulnar vein
CC. vertebral vein

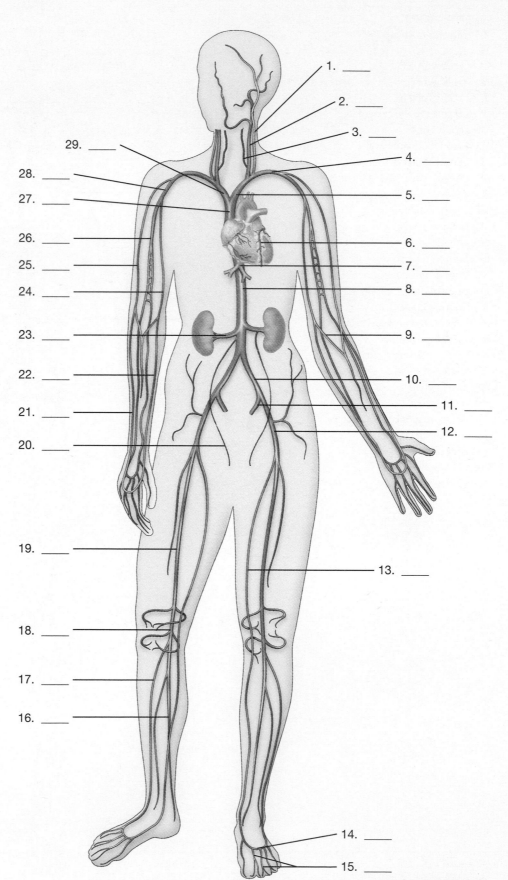

1. _____
2. _____
3. _____
4. _____
5. _____
6. _____
7. _____
8. _____
9. _____
10. _____
11. _____
12. _____
13. _____
14. _____
15. _____
16. _____
17. _____
18. _____
19. _____
20. _____
21. _____
22. _____
23. _____
24. _____
25. _____
26. _____
27. _____
28. _____
29. _____

© *Body Scientific International*

Section 12.4 Vocabulary Review I

Match each vocabulary word with its definition.

A. aneurysm
B. angina pectoris
C. atherosclerosis
D. brachial artery
E. cardiomyopathy
F. carotid artery
G. cerebrovascular accident
H. coronary artery disease
I. hypertension
J. peripheral vascular disease
K. radial artery
L. transient ischemic attack (TIA)

_____ 1. narrowing of the arteries in the legs
_____ 2. severe pain due to lack of blood supply to the heart
_____ 3. artery in the arm
_____ 4. temporary lack of blood flow to the brain
_____ 5. artery located in the neck
_____ 6. plaque buildup in arteries supplying oxygenated blood to the heart
_____ 7. hardening of the arteries
_____ 8. disease that weakens the heart muscle
_____ 9. part of an artery balloons out and may rupture
_____ 10. high blood pressure
_____ 11. artery on thumb side of wrist
_____ 12. stroke

Section 12.4 Vocabulary Review II

Match each vocabulary word with its definition.

A. atrial fibrillation
B. bradycardia
C. dysrhythmia
D. endocarditis
E. heart block
F. heart murmur
G. ischemia
H. mitral valve prolapse
I. myocardial infarction
J. myocarditis
K. palpitations
L. pericarditis
M. premature atrial contraction (PAC)
N. premature ventricular contraction (PVC)
O. tachycardia
P. valvular stenosis
Q. ventricular fibrillation
R. ventricular tachycardia

_____ 1. sensations of a rapid heartbeat
_____ 2. heartbeat less than 60 beats/minute
_____ 3. heart attack

_____ 4. lack of blood flow
_____ 5. condition in which the ventricles quiver rather than beat
_____ 6. inflammation of the middle layer of the heart
_____ 7. delay or blockage of impulses from the SA node
_____ 8. abnormal heart sound
_____ 9. irregular heartbeat
_____ 10. heart rate more than 100 beats/minute
_____ 11. condition in which the atria contract too soon
_____ 12. inflammation of the innermost layer of the heart
_____ 13. condition in which the bicuspid valve does not close properly
_____ 14. inflammation of the sac around the heart
_____ 15. rapid beating of the ventricles
_____ 16. condition in which the atria quiver rather than beat
_____ 17. condition in which the ventricles contract too soon
_____ 18. narrowing of heart valves

Section 12.4 Study Questions

1. How do you check a person's pulse?
2. What is the procedure for measuring a patient's blood pressure?
3. What is the basic formula for calculating BMI?
4. What does each of the deflection waves in an ECG represent?
5. Name and describe two valve abnormalities.
6. What is an aneurysm?
7. What are the long-term effects of atherosclerosis?
8. What is a myocardial infarction?
9. What are the risk factors for hypertension?
10. What is a cerebrovascular accident?

Medical Terminology

For each item, identify the word parts and their meanings, and then provide the meaning of the medical term. Use a medical dictionary or the textbook if you need help.

1. cardiomegaly

   root/combining form: _____

   meaning: _____

   root/combining form: _____

   meaning: _____

   suffix: _____

   meaning: _____

   meaning of word: _____

Name: _____   Date: _____

2. vasculitis

    root/combining form: _____

    meaning: _____

    suffix: _____

    meaning: _____

    meaning of word: _____

3. cardiomyopathy

    root/combining form: _____

    meaning: _____

    root/combining form: _____

    meaning: _____

    suffix: _____

    meaning: _____

    meaning of word: _____

4. pulmonary

    root/combining form: _____

    meaning: _____

    suffix: _____

    meaning: _____

    meaning of word: _____

5. cardioplegia

    root/combining form: _____

    meaning: _____

    suffix: _____

    meaning: _____

    meaning of word: _____

6. ventriculopleural

    root/combining form: _____

    meaning: _____

    root/combining form: _____

    meaning: _____

    suffix: _____

    meaning: _____

    meaning of word: _____

7. arteriopathy

    root/combining form: _____

    meaning: _____

    suffix: _____

    meaning: _____

    meaning of word: _____

8. vasomotor

    root/combining form: _____

    meaning: _____

    suffix: _____

    meaning: _____

    meaning of word: _____

9. pulmonology

    root/combining form: _____

    meaning: _____

    suffix: _____

    meaning: _____

    meaning of word: _____

10. atriomegaly

    root/combining form: _____

    meaning: _____

    suffix: _____

    meaning: _____

    meaning of word: _____

13 The Lymphatic and Immune Systems

Name: _____   Date: _____

Section 13.1 Vocabulary Review

Match each vocabulary word with its definition.

A. B lymphocytes (B cells)
B. endothelial cells
C. interstitial fluid
D. lingual tonsils
E. lymph
F. lymph nodes
G. lymphatic nodules
H. lymphatic trunks
I. lymphatic valves
J. lymphatic vessels
K. lymphocytes
L. macrophages
M. mucosa-associated lymphatic tissue (MALT)
N. natural killer (NK) cells
O. palatine tonsils
P. pathogens
Q. pharyngeal tonsil
R. spleen
S. T lymphocytes (T cells)

_____ 1. inner lining of lymphatic vessels

_____ 2. two areas of lymphatic tissue at the back of the mouth

_____ 3. cause diseases

_____ 4. interstitial fluid within lymph vessels

_____ 5. matured in the thymus

_____ 6. "swollen glands"

_____ 7. largest lymphatic organ

_____ 8. fluid between cells

_____ 9. adenoids

_____ 10. lymphatic tissue that guards entrances to the body

_____ 11. produce antibodies

_____ 12. flaps to prevent lymph from flowing backward

_____ 13. includes B and T cells

_____ 14. two areas of lymphatic tissue at the base of the tongue

_____ 15. ductwork that carries lymph

_____ 16. lymphocytes that destroy virus-infected cells and cancer cells

_____ 17. small clusters of tissue formed by lymphocytes and macrophages

_____ 18. cells that engulf foreign invaders

_____ 19. large lymph vessels that drain lymph

Section 13.1 Study Questions

1. What are the three main functions of the lymphatic system?

2. Name the elements of the lymphatic system.

3. What are the major lymphatic vessels?

4. List and describe the functions of the different types of lymphocytes.

5. What is meant by the term *MALT*?

6. Where are the different types of tonsils located?

7. Describe the structure of a lymph node

8. What are the spleen's lymphatic functions?

9. How do the red pulp and white pulp in the spleen differ?

10. What is the immune function of the thymus?

Section 13.1 Labeling
The Lymphatic System

Identify the structures of the lymphatic system.

Labeling Terms

A. appendix
B. axillary lymph node
C. cervical lymph node
D. cisterna chyli
E. inguinal lymph node

F. lumbar lymph node
G. pelvic lymph node
H. red bone marrow
I. right lymphatic duct

J. spleen
K. thoracic duct
L. thymus gland
M. tonsils

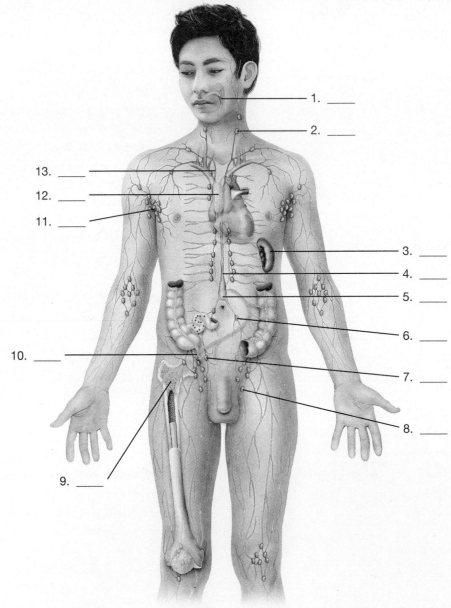

1. _____
2. _____
13. _____
12. _____
11. _____
3. _____
4. _____
5. _____
6. _____
10. _____
7. _____
8. _____
9. _____

© Body Scientific International

Lymphatic Ducts and Vessels

Identify the lymphatic ducts and vessels.

Labeling Terms

A. azygos vein (draining vein)
B. cisterna chyli
C. diaphragm
D. hemiazygos vein (draining vein)
E. internal jugular veins
F. intestinal trunk

G. left broncho-mediastinal trunk
H. left jugular trunk
I. left lumbar trunk
J. left subclavian trunk
K. right broncho-mediastinal trunk
L. right jugular trunk

M. right lumbar trunk
N. right lymphatic duct
O. right subclavian trunk
P. thoracic duct
Q. thoracic lymph nodes

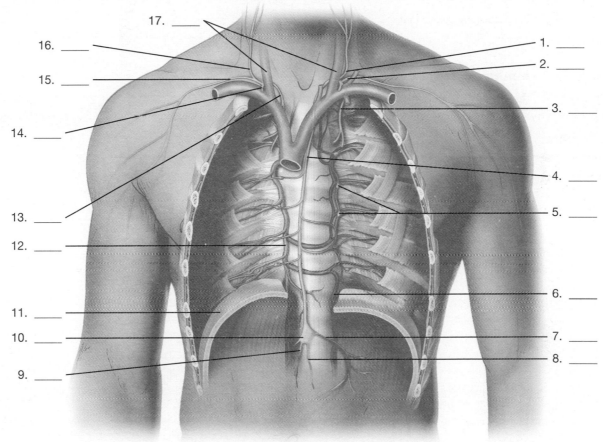

17. ____
16. ____
15. ____
14. ____
13. ____
12. ____
11. ____
10. ____
9. ____

1. ____
2. ____
3. ____
4. ____
5. ____
6. ____
7. ____
8. ____

© Body Scientific International

Section 13.2 Vocabulary Review

Match each vocabulary word with its definition.

A. alternative pathway
B. classical pathway
C. complement proteins
D. complement system
E. exocytosis
F. fever
G. inflammatory response
H. interferons
I. lectin pathway

J. mast cells
K. monocytes
L. neutrophils
M. opsonins
N. phagocytes
O. phagocytosis
P. prostaglandins
Q. pyrogens

_____ 1. higher than normal body temperature

_____ 2. fatty acids that affect body temperature and inflammation

_____ 3. process in which the C3 protein binds directly to bacteria

_____ 4. process in which the membrane of a phagocytic vesicle fuses with the phagocyte's membrane

_____ 5. most common white blood cells

_____ 6. proteins released from cells that interfere with the reproduction of viruses

_____ 7. cells that release histamine

_____ 8. process in which a C1 protein interacts with an antibody

_____ 9. process of a WBC engulfing and digesting foreign material

_____ 10. process in which lectin binds to a sugar molecule on bacteria

_____ 11. proteins that make cells more attractive to phagocytes

_____ 12. proteins that work with cells and antibodies to defend the body from infections

_____ 13. large WBCs that become phagocytes

_____ 14. swelling, redness, and pain in damaged tissues

_____ 15. cells that engulf and digest foreign material

_____ 16. involves more than 30 proteins that work together to destroy foreign material

_____ 17. chemicals that bring about a fever

Section 13.2 Study Questions

1. How does the skin participate in immunity?

2. What is phagocytosis?

3. Which types of white blood cells participate in phagocytosis?

4. What are natural killer cells?

5. Describe the classical pathway in the complement system.

6. How is the lectin pathway different from the classical pathway?

7. What is the alternative pathway?

8. How does interferon function?

9. How do mast cells participate in the inflammatory response?

10. How does a fever contribute to immunity?

Section 13.2 Labeling
The Skin and Its Structures

Identify the structures present in the skin.

Labeling terms

A. artery
B. dermis
C. duct of sweat gland
D. epidermis
E. fatty tissue

F. hair follicle
G. hair shaft
H. lymphatic vessel
I. nerve

J. sebaceous gland
K. subcutaneous tissue
L. sweat gland
M. vein

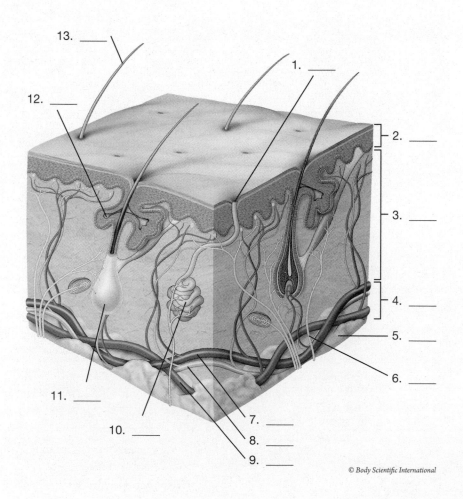

13. _____
12. _____
1. _____
2. _____
3. _____
4. _____
5. _____
6. _____
11. _____
10. _____
7. _____
8. _____
9. _____

© Body Scientific International

Section 13.3 Vocabulary Review

Match each vocabulary word with its definition.

A. active immunity
B. antibody-mediated immunity
C. antigen-presenting cells (APCs)
D. apoptosis
E. cell-mediated immunity
F. clonal selection
G. immune system
H. immunoglobulins
I. major histocompatibility complex glycoproteins (MHCs)
J. memory cells
K. passive immunity
L. precipitation
M. primary immune response
N. secondary immune response

_____ 1. self-destruction of cells

_____ 2. initial immune response to a foreign invader

_____ 3. clumping together of antigens and antibodies

_____ 4. humoral immunity

_____ 5. cellular immunity

_____ 6. all the cells and chemicals that defend the body against disease

_____ 7. immune response when the body encounters a foreign invader that it has seen before

_____ 8. process in which lymphocytes make exact copies of themselves

_____ 9. getting antibodies from an outside source

_____ 10. antibody-mediated immunity in which the body's own cells make antibodies

_____ 11. cells that process antigens and present them in a form that lymphocytes can recognize

_____ 12. B and T cells that recognize something foreign that they have encountered before

_____ 13. antibodies

_____ 14. proteins on the surface of WBCs that help to distinguish between self and nonself

Section 13.3 Study Questions

1. What occurs when a patient has severe combined immune deficiency (SCID)?

2. What is an antigen?

3. How does apoptosis protect the body?

4. How do Class I MHC proteins and Class II MHC proteins differ?

5. What are antibodies?

6. Describe what is meant by *active immunity*.

7. What is passive immunity?

8. List the five major classes of antibodies.

9. Explain how a secondary immune response works.

10. What is cell-mediated immunity?

Section 13.4 Vocabulary Review

Match each vocabulary word with its definition.

A. acquired immunodeficiency syndrome (AIDS)
B. allergen
C. allergen immunotherapy
D. anaphylaxis
E. autoimmune disorder
F. human immunodeficiency virus (HIV)
G. immunosuppression
H. lymphedema
I. metastasis
J. opportunistic infection
K. tolerance

_____ 1. condition in which an allergic response lessens or goes away entirely

_____ 2. disease in which patients have a weakened immune system due to an HIV infection

_____ 3. swelling due to accumulated lymph

_____ 4. an infection that may target an individual with a weak immune system

_____ 5. allergy shots

_____ 6. the virus that causes AIDS

_____ 7. a substance that brings about an inappropriate immune response

_____ 8. process of cancer spreading to other locations in the body

_____ 9. life-threatening allergic response

_____ 10. condition in which the body attacks its own tissue

_____ 11. reduction in the functioning of the immune system

Section 13.4 Study Questions

1. How do lymph nodes help to detect whether cancer has metastasized?

2. What is an allergen?

3. Why does anaphylaxis sometimes occur as a result of an allergy?

4. What is the purpose of allergen immunotherapy?

5. Why is an individual who has received an organ transplant more susceptible than other people to infections?

6. What are autoimmune disorders?

7. List three examples of autoimmune disorders.

8. How is the HIV virus transmitted?

9. What are the symptoms of an HIV infection?

10. Why are opportunistic infections often the way that AIDS is diagnosed?

Medical Terminology

For each item, identify the word parts and their meanings, and then provide the meaning of the medical term. Use a medical dictionary or the textbook if you need help.

1. lymphangiogram

   root/combining form: _____

   meaning: _____

   root/combining form: _____

   meaning: _____

   suffix: _____

   meaning: _____

   meaning of word: _____

2. melanoderma

   root/combining form: _____

   meaning: _____

   suffix: _____

   meaning: _____

   meaning of word: _____

3. lymphadenopathy

   root/combining form: _____

   meaning: _____

   root/combining form: _____

   meaning: _____

   suffix: _____

   meaning: _____

   meaning of word: _____

4. melanoma

   root/combining form: _____

   meaning: _____

   suffix: _____

   meaning: _____

   meaning of word: _____

5. lymphadenitis

   root/combining form: _____

   meaning: _____

   root/combining form: _____

   meaning: _____

   suffix: _____

   meaning: _____

   meaning of word: _____

6. melanosis

   root/combining form: _____

   meaning: _____

   suffix: _____

   meaning: _____

   meaning of word: _____

7. agglutinogen

   root/combining form: _____

   meaning: _____

   suffix: _____

   meaning: _____

   meaning of word: _____

8. splenomegaly

   root/combining form: _____

   meaning: _____

   suffix: _____

   meaning: _____

   meaning of word: _____

9. dysphagia

    prefix: _____

    meaning: _____

    root/combining form: _____

    meaning: _____

    suffix: _____

    meaning: _____

    meaning of word: _____

10. pyrolysis

    root/combining form: _____

    meaning: _____

    suffix: _____

    meaning: _____

    meaning of word: _____

NOTES

14 The Digestive System and Metabolism

Name: _____ Date: _____

Section 14.1 Vocabulary Review

Match each vocabulary word with its definition.

A. anabolism
B. basal metabolic rate (BMR)
C. calorie
D. catabolism
E. energy
F. metabolism

_____ 1. combining of small molecules to form larger molecules

_____ 2. capacity to do work

_____ 3. heat required to raise the temperature of 1 kilogram of water by 1°C

_____ 4. breakdown of large molecules into smaller ones

_____ 5. energy needed to sustain metabolism while at rest for one day

_____ 6. all of the chemical reactions that occur in the body cells

Section 14.1 Study Questions

1. How do chemical, kinetic, and potential energy differ?

2. What is a Calorie, and what does it measure?

3. Describe metabolism.

4. Compare and contrast the terms *anabolism* and *catabolism*.

5. Describe the process by which carbohydrates are broken down and ATP is generated.

6. How many molecules of ATP are generated from the complete breakdown of one molecule of glucose?

7. What is gluconeogenesis?

8. What is glycogenolysis?

9. When and how are triglycerides formed?

10. What factors can affect a person's basal metabolic rate?

Section 14.2 Vocabulary Review

Match each vocabulary word with its definition.

A. coenzymes
B. enzyme
C. lipids
D. macronutrients
E. micronutrients
F. minerals
G. monounsaturated fats
H. nutrients
I. polyunsaturated fats
J. trans-unsaturated fats
K. vitamin deficiency
L. vitamins

_____ 1. minerals and vitamins that are needed in small amounts by the body

_____ 2. artificially produced fatty acids

_____ 3. substance that speeds up a reaction

_____ 4. minerals and vitamins that are needed in large amounts by the body

_____ 5. long-term lack of an organic chemical in the body needed for metabolism

_____ 6. includes corn and soybean oil

_____ 7. includes canola and olive oil

_____ 8. molecule necessary for an enzyme to work

_____ 9. chemicals needed for energy, growth, and maintenance

_____ 10. fats

_____ 11. elements the body needs in small amounts, such as calcium and phosphorus

_____ 12. organic chemicals needed by the body

Section 14.2 Study Questions

1. What percentage of a person's diet should be carbohydrates?

2. What is the recommended percentage of proteins in a person's diet?

3. Name the nine amino acids that the body cannot produce in sufficient amounts.

4. List four overall diet recommendations to lose weight.

5. Which types of lipids do experts urge people to limit in their diet?

6. What might happen if you took too many water-soluble vitamins? Fat-soluble vitamins?

7. What is the main function of most water-soluble vitamins?

8. What health problems may occur in a person who has a deficiency of vitamin D?

9. Which mineral is key in transporting oxygen in the blood?

10. Why do some health experts recommend reducing your salt intake?

Section 14.3 Vocabulary Review

Match each vocabulary word with its definition.

A. absorption
B. alimentary canal
C. chemical breakdown
D. chyme
E. colon
F. defecation
G. emulsification
H. esophagus
I. gallbladder
J. gastrointestinal (GI) tract
K. gingiva
L. ingestion
M. large intestine
N. mechanical breakdown
O. propulsion
P. rectum
Q. small intestine
R. stomach

_____ 1. structure used for short-term feces storage

_____ 2. stores and concentrates bile

_____ 3. food mixed with gastric juice in the stomach

_____ 4. movement of nutrients from the small intestine into the blood

_____ 5. contains an additional muscle layer to help churn food

_____ 6. intake of food into the mouth

_____ 7. movement of food through the GI tract

_____ 8. gums

_____ 9. physical breaking of food into smaller pieces

_____ 10. gastrointestinal tract

_____ 11. dividing a large glob of fat into smaller pieces

_____ 12. located between the pharynx and the stomach

_____ 13. part of the GI tract where the most digestion and food absorption takes place

_____ 14. longest part of the large intestine

_____ 15. getting rid of feces

_____ 16. breakdown of food by enzymes

_____ 17. alimentary canal

_____ 18. includes the cecum and colon

Section 14.3 Study Questions

1. What are the accessory structures that contribute to digestion?

2. Describe the layers of the GI tract.

3. What structure holds a tooth's root securely in its socket?

4. What are the chemical and mechanical activities that take place in the mouth?

5. Why is the presence of hydrochloric acid advantageous in the stomach?

6. Describe the chemical and mechanical events that occur in the stomach.

7. What is the digestive function of the liver?

8. What are the digestive components of pancreatic juice?

9. What substances are absorbed in the small intestine?

10. What is the function of the bacteria in the large intestine?

Section 14.3 Labeling
Organs of the Digestive System

Identify the organs of the digestive system.

Labeling Terms

A. anus
B. esophagus
C. gallbladder
D. large intestine

E. liver
F. mouth
G. pancreas
H. parotid

I. pharynx
J. rectum
K. salivary glands
L. small intestine

M. stomach
N. sublingual
O. submandibular

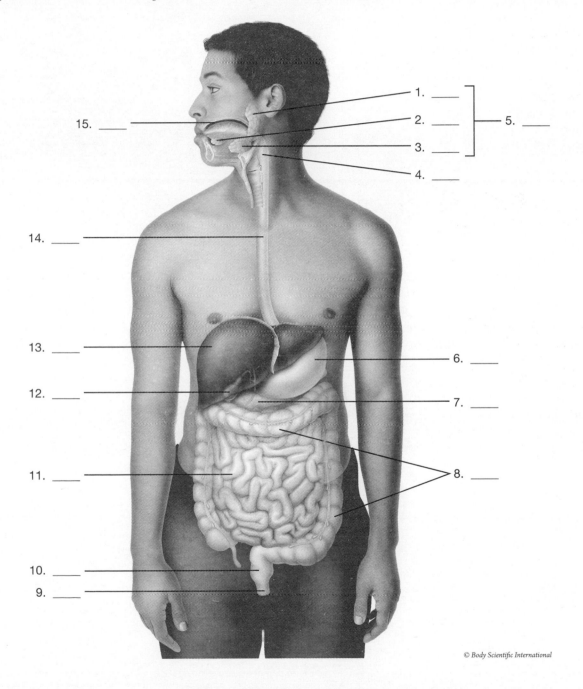

© Body Scientific International

The Stomach

Identify the structures of the stomach.

Labeling Terms

A. anterior surface
B. body
C. cardia
D. circular muscle layer
E. duodenum of small intestine
F. esophagus
G. fundus
H. greater curvature
I. lesser curvature
J. longitudinal muscle layer
K. oblique muscle layer
L. pyloric region
M. pyloric sphincter
N. pylorus
O. rugae

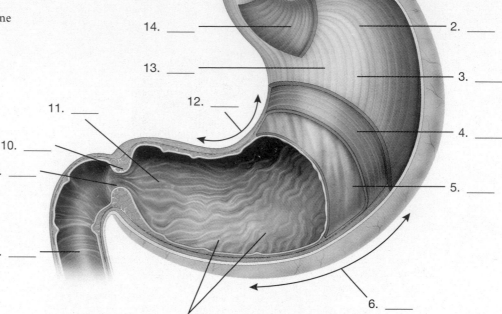

15. _____   1. _____
14. _____   2. _____
13. _____   3. _____
12. _____   4. _____
11. _____   5. _____
10. _____   6. _____
9. _____   7. _____
8. _____

© Body Scientific International

The Small Intestine

Identify the structures of the small intestine.

Labeling Terms

A. ascending colon
B. cecum
C. descending colon
D. duodenum
E. ileum
F. jejunum
G. rectum
H. sigmoid colon
I. transverse colon (cut)

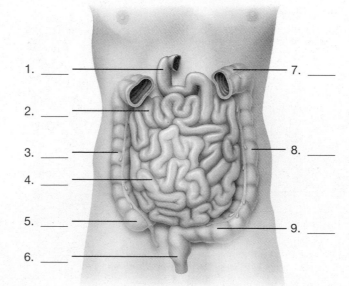

1. _____   7. _____
2. _____   8. _____
3. _____   9. _____
4. _____
5. _____
6. _____

© Body Scientific International

The Liver, Gallbladder, Pancreas, and Duodenum

Identify the digestive structures.

Labeling Terms

A. common bile duct
B. common bile sphincter
C. common hepatic duct
D. cystic duct
E. duodenal papilla
F. duodenum
G. gallbladder
H. hepatopancreatic ampulla and sphincter
I. jejunum
J. left hepatic duct
K. left lobe of the liver
L. pancreas
M. pancreatic duct
N. pancreatic sphincter
O. right hepatic duct
P. right lobe of liver

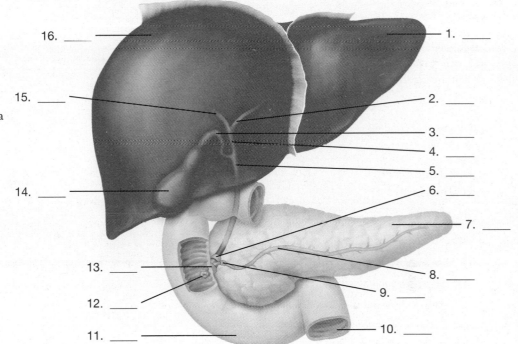

16. _____   1. _____
15. _____   2. _____
14. _____   3. _____
13. _____   4. _____
12. _____   5. _____
11. _____   6. _____
             7. _____
             8. _____
             9. _____
             10. _____

© Body Scientific International

The Large Intestine

Identify the parts of the large intestine.

Labeling Terms

A. anal canal
B. appendix
C. ascending colon
D. cecum
E. cut end of ileum
F. descending colon
G. external anal sphincter
H. ileocecal valve
I. rectum
J. sigmoid colon
K. transverse colon

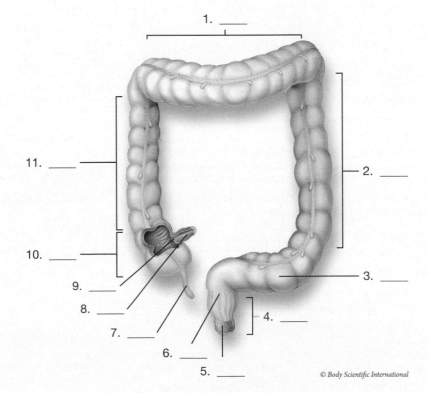

1. _____
2. _____
3. _____
4. _____
5. _____
6. _____
7. _____
8. _____
9. _____
10. _____
11. _____

© Body Scientific International

Section 14.4 Vocabulary Review

Match each vocabulary word with its definition.

A. cholecystectomy
B. constipation
C. Crohn's disease
D. diarrhea
E. gallstones
F. gastroenteritis
G. gastroesophageal reflux
H. gastroesophageal reflux disease (GERD)
I. hepatitis
J. inflammatory bowel disease
K. pancreatitis
L. peptic ulcer
M. periodontal disease
N. ulcerative colitis

_____ 1. watery feces

_____ 2. solid crystals in the gallbladder

_____ 3. removal of the gallbladder

_____ 4. inflammation of the liver, usually caused by a virus

_____ 5. disease of the gums and teeth

_____ 6. lack of water in feces

_____ 7. condition in which gastric juice enters the esophagus

_____ 8. chronic disease that causes the small intestine and colon to be inflamed

_____ 9. spot of the mucosa in the stomach, duodenum, or esophagus is worn away

_____ 10. chronically inflamed lower esophagus

_____ 11. inflammation of the pancreas

_____ 12. inflammation of the stomach or intestine that results in pain and vomiting

_____ 13. chronic inflammation of the walls of the small and large intestines

_____ 14. inflammation of the colon and intestinal mucosa

Section 14.4 Study Questions

1. What health effects could develop from untreated gingivitis?

2. What can people who have gastroesophageal reflux disease (GERD) do to relieve their symptoms?

3. What causes a peptic ulcer?

4. How is gastroenteritis treated?

5. What are the physical effects of Crohn's disease?

6. How does the time feces stay in the large intestine relate to diarrhea and constipation?

7. Describe the symptoms of hepatitis.

8. What causes pancreatitis?

9. What are gallstones, and where do they commonly lodge?

10. What is the most common method of identifying colon cancer and other digestive diseases that affect the intestines?

Medical Terminology

For each item, identify the word parts and their meanings, and then provide the meaning of the medical term. Use a medical dictionary or the textbook if you need help.

1. hepatomegaly

   root/combining form: _____

   meaning: _____

   suffix: _____

   meaning: _____

   meaning of word: _____

2. hypoglycemia

   prefix: _____

   meaning: _____

   root/combining form: _____

   meaning: _____

   suffix: _____

   meaning: _____

   meaning of word: _____

3. hepatology

   root/combining form: _____

   meaning: _____

   suffix: _____

   meaning: _____

   meaning of word: _____

4. proteinuria

   root/combining form: _____

   meaning: _____

   root/combining form: _____

   meaning: _____

   suffix: _____

   meaning: _____

   meaning of word: _____

5. cholangitis

    root/combining form: _____

    meaning: _____

    suffix: _____

    meaning: _____

    meaning of word: _____

6. hepatotoxic

    root/combining form: _____

    meaning: _____

    root/combining form: _____

    meaning: _____

    suffix: _____

    meaning: _____

    meaning of word: _____

7. myelomeningocele

    root/combining form: _____

    meaning: _____

    root/combining form: _____

    meaning: _____

    suffix: _____

    meaning: _____

    meaning of word: _____

8. cholangiography

    root/combining form: _____

    meaning: _____

    root/combining form: _____

    meaning: _____

    suffix: _____

    meaning: _____

    meaning of word: _____

9. hepatoblastoma

    root/combining form: _____

    meaning: _____

    suffix: _____

    meaning: _____

    meaning of word: _____

10. hemangioma

    root/combining form: _____

    meaning: _____

    root/combining form: _____

    meaning: _____

    suffix: _____

    meaning: _____

    meaning of word: _____

NOTES

15 The Urinary System

Name: _____ Date: _____

Section 15.1 Vocabulary Review

Match each vocabulary word with its definition.

A. collecting duct
B. distal convoluted tubule
C. glomerulus
D. nephron
E. nephron loop
F. proximal convoluted tubule (PCT)
G. renal corpuscle
H. renal cortex
I. renal medulla
J. renal pelvis
K. renal tubule
L. urinary system
M. vasa recta

_____ 1. cluster of capillaries surrounded by the glomerular capsule

_____ 2. regulates the body's internal environment by controlling excretions

_____ 3. microscopic units within the kidney that form urine

_____ 4. part of a nephron between the glomerular capsule and the nephron loop

_____ 5. large collecting area within the kidney just before urine enters the ureter

_____ 6. tube that collects urine from several nephrons

_____ 7. the glomerulus and its surrounding glomerular capsule

_____ 8. outer portion of the kidney

_____ 9. blood vessels located near the nephron loops

_____ 10. inner portion of the kidney

_____ 11. part of a nephron that leads to a collecting duct

_____ 12. U-shaped portion of a nephron

_____ 13. part of nephron that goes from the glomerular capsule to the collecting duct

Section 15.1 Study Questions

1. How do the kidneys help maintain homeostasis in the body?

2. Name three functions of the kidneys that are unrelated to excretion.

3. What is the external appearance of the kidney?

4. What are the two main areas within the kidneys, and how do they differ?

5. What is the basic working unit of the kidney?

6. Name the two main parts of a nephron.

7. Describe the structure of the renal corpuscle.

8. Trace the path of filtrate through the renal tubule.

9. How do cortical and juxtamedullary nephrons differ?

10. Describe the blood flow from the heart through the kidney and back to the heart.

Section 15.1 Labeling
Urinary System Anatomy

Identify the components of the urinary system.

Labeling Terms

A. abdominal aorta
B. adrenal gland
C. esophagus (cut)
D. hepatic veins (cut)
E. inferior vena cava
F. kidney
G. rectum (cut)
H. renal artery
I. renal hilum
J. renal vein
K. ureter
L. urethra
M. urinary bladder
N. uterus (part of female reproductive system)

1. _____
2. _____
3. _____
4. _____
5. _____
6. _____
7. _____
8. _____
9. _____
10. _____
11. _____
12. _____
13. _____
14. _____

© Body Scientific International

The Kidney

Identify the structures of the kidney.

Labeling Terms

A. fibrous capsule
B. hilum
C. papilla of pyramid
D. renal column
E. renal cortex
F. renal medulla
G. renal pelvis
H. renal pyramid
   in renal medulla
I. ureter

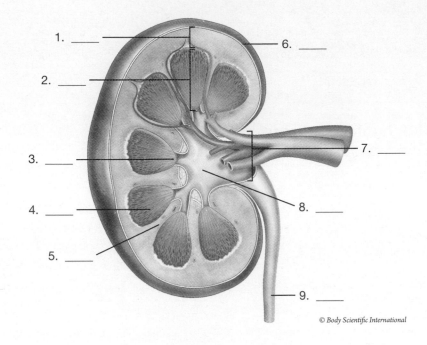

1. ____   6. ____
2. ____
3. ____   7. ____
4. ____   8. ____
5. ____   9. ____

© Body Scientific International

The Nephron

Identify the components of a nephron.

Labeling Terms

A. afferent arteriole
B. collecting duct
C. descending limb
   of nephron loop
D. distal convoluted
   tubule (DCT)
E. efferent arteriole
F. nephron loop
G. peritubular capillaries
H. proximal convoluted
   tubule (PCT)
I. renal cortex
J. renal medulla
K. thick ascending limb
   of the nephron loop
L. thin ascending limb
   of the nephron loop
M. vasa recta

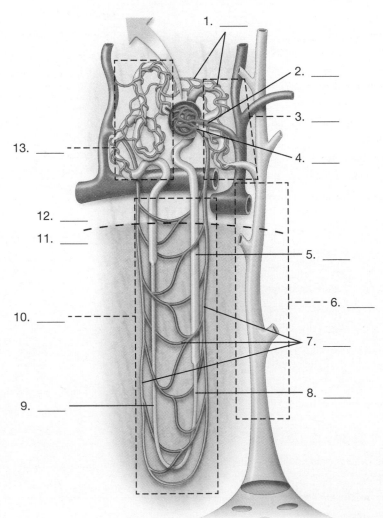

1. ____
2. ____
3. ____
4. ____
5. ____
6. ____
7. ____
8. ____
9. ____
10. ____
11. ____
12. ____
13. ____

© Body Scientific International

Section 15.2 Vocabulary Review

Match each vocabulary word with its definition.

A. aldosterone
B. angiotensin
C. antidiuretic hormone (ADH)
D. atrial natriuretic peptide (ANP)
E. detrusor
F. diuresis
G. external urethral sphincter
H. glomerular filtration
I. glomerular filtration rate (GFR)
J. hydrostatic pressure
K. internal urethral sphincter
L. micturition
M. osmosis
N. osmotic pressure
O. reabsorption
P. renin
Q. secretion
R. trigone
S. ureter
T. urethra
U. urinary bladder

_____ 1. structure that stores urine before it is expelled from the body

_____ 2. muscle that makes up part of the bladder wall

_____ 3. urinating

_____ 4. region with triangular borders: two ureteric orifices and one urethral orifice

_____ 5. hormone from the pituitary gland that helps to conserve water during urine formation

_____ 6. stage of urine formation where substances travel from the glomerulus into the glomerular capsule

_____ 7. tube that goes from the bladder to outside the body

_____ 8. stage of urine formation in which substances travel back into the bloodstream

_____ 9. enzyme made by the kidneys to help make angiotensin

_____ 10. hormone from the heart that lowers blood pressure

_____ 11. tube from each kidney to the bladder

_____ 12. amount of fluid per time that goes from the glomerulus to the glomerular capsule

_____ 13. making urine

_____ 14. smooth muscle around the opening at the bottom of the bladder

_____ 15. increases when the amount of dissolved substances in water increases

_____ 16. hormone that increases blood pressure by constricting blood vessels

_____ 17. stage of urine formation in which substances move from the blood into the nephron

_____ 18. hormone made in the adrenal cortex that conserves water during urine formation

_____ 19. skeletal muscle around the urethra to control urination

_____ 20. pushes water from areas of high pressure to low pressure

_____ 21. movement of water from an area of high water concentration to an area of low water concentration

Section 15.2 Study Questions

1. Name the three stages of urine formation.
2. What is the importance of the filtration membrane?
3. What events happen during glomerular filtration?
4. How does hydrostatic pressure influence glomerular filtration?
5. What occurs during the reabsorption phase of urine formation?
6. What events occur during the secretion phase of urine formation?
7. What is the countercurrent mechanism?
8. Briefly discuss how the hormones aldosterone, atrial natriuretic peptide, and antidiuretic hormone regulate the formation of urine.
9. Describe the physical location and arrangement of the ureters, bladder, and urethra.
10. Describe the process of micturition.

Section 15.2 Labeling
The Renal Medulla

Identify the components of the renal medulla.

Labeling Terms

A. collecting duct
B. descending limb of the nephron loop
C. interstitial fluid
D. nephron loop
E. thick ascending limb of the nephron loop
F. thin ascending limb of the nephron loop
G. vasa recta

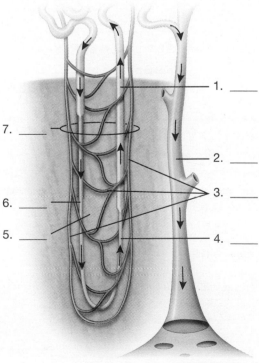

1. _____
2. _____
3. _____
4. _____
5. _____
6. _____
7. _____

© *Body Scientific International*

The Male and Female Bladder and Urethra

Identify the structures within the male and female bladder and urethra.

Labeling Terms

A. bladder neck
B. detrusor muscle
C. external urethral orifice
D. external urethral sphincter
E. intermediate part of the urethra

F. internal urethral sphincter
G. peritoneum
H. prostate
I. prostatic urethra
J. rugae

K. trigone of bladder
L. ureteral orifices
M. ureter
N. urethra
O. urogenital diaphragm

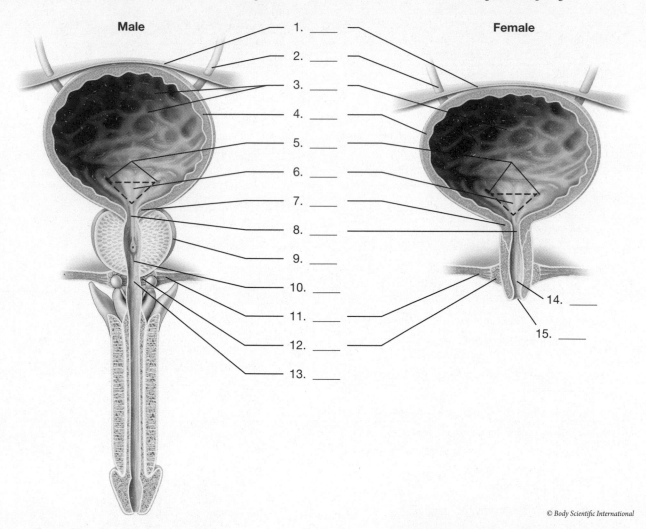

Male   **Female**

1. ____
2. ____
3. ____
4. ____
5. ____
6. ____
7. ____
8. ____
9. ____
10. ____
11. ____
12. ____
13. ____

14. ____
15. ____

© Body Scientific International

Section 15.3 Vocabulary Review

Match each vocabulary word with its definition.

A. chronic kidney disease
B. creatinine
C. hemodialysis
D. kidney stone
E. osmotic diuresis
F. peritoneal dialysis

G. renal dialysis
H. urine specific gravity
I. urinalysis
J. urinary tract
   infection (UTI)

____ 1. infection in the urinary system, usually from bacteria entering the urethra

____ 2. blood travels through a machine for filtration and returned to patient

____ 3. byproduct of muscle movement

____ 4. uses the peritoneum to filter the blood

____ 5. solid mass in the kidney

____ 6. calculated by dividing the density of a urine sample by the density of water

____ 7. examination of urine in the laboratory

____ 8. long-term filtration rate of less than 60 mL per minute

____ 9. increased production of urine to osmotic pressure levels

____ 10. removing toxins from the blood via artificial means

Copyright Goodheart-Willcox Co., Inc.
May not be reproduced or posted to a publicly accessible website.

Section 15.3 Study Questions

1. What are the physical characteristics of normal urine?

2. What is the chemical composition of urine?

3. How is the glomerular filtration rate determined, and what does its value tell the examiner?

4. Why do the two diseases diabetes mellitus and diabetes insipidus both start with the term *diabetes*?

5. What is diabetes mellitus, and how is it treated?

6. What is diabetes insipidus, and how is it treated?

7. How do hemodialysis and peritoneal dialysis differ?

8. What are kidney stones, and what are the treatment options?

9. How do stress incontinence and urge incontinence differ?

10. Why do females have more urinary tract infections than men?

Medical Terminology

For each item, identify the word parts and their meanings, and then provide the meaning of the medical term. Use a medical dictionary or the textbook if you need help.

1. cystoscopy

    root/combining form: _____

    meaning: _____

    suffix: _____

    meaning: _____

    meaning of word: _____

2. retropharyngeal

    prefix: _____

    meaning: _____

    root/combining form: _____

    meaning: _____

    suffix: _____

    meaning: _____

    meaning of word: _____

3. juxtavesicular

    prefix: _____

    meaning: _____

    root/combining form: _____

    meaning: _____

    suffix: _____

    meaning: _____

    meaning of word: _____

4. retropubic prostatectomy

    prefix: _____

    meaning: _____

    root/combining form: _____

    meaning: _____

    suffix: _____

    meaning: _____

    root/combining form: _____

    meaning: _____

    suffix: _____

    meaning: _____

    meaning of word: _____

5. lithotomy

    root/combining form: _____

    meaning: _____

    suffix: _____

    meaning: _____

    meaning of word: _____

6. nephrolithiasis

    root/combining form: _____

    meaning: _____

    root/combining form: _____

    meaning: _____

    suffix: _____

    meaning: _____

    meaning of word: _____

7. cystometry

    root/combining form: _____

    meaning: _____

    suffix: _____

    meaning: _____

    meaning of word: _____

8. amenorrhea

    prefix: _____

    meaning: _____

    root/combining form: _____

    meaning: _____

    suffix: _____

    meaning: _____

    meaning of word: _____

9. natriuresis

    root/combining form: _____

    meaning: _____

    root/combining form: _____

    meaning: _____

    suffix: _____

    meaning: _____

    meaning of word: _____

10. urethroplasty

    root/combining form: _____

    meaning: _____

    suffix: _____

    meaning: _____

    meaning of word: _____

16 The Male and Female Reproductive Systems

Name: _____ Date: _____

Section 16.1 Vocabulary Review

Match each vocabulary word with its definition.

A. centromere
B. chromatids
C. chromosomes
D. crossovers
E. diploid
F. fertilization
G. follicle stimulating hormone (FSH)
H. gametes
I. haploid
J. luteinizing hormone (LH)
K. meiosis
L. menarche
M. zygote

_____ 1. connection between homologous chromosomes

_____ 2. beginning of menstruation

_____ 3. cell division that produces sperm and ova

_____ 4. point at which two sister chromatids join

_____ 5. having the normal number of chromosomes from two parents

_____ 6. result of the union of a sperm and an egg

_____ 7. hormone that causes ovulation in females

_____ 8. paired strands of a duplicated chromosome

_____ 9. having half of the normal number of chromosomes

_____ 10. the process of sperm and egg uniting to form offspring

_____ 11. structures in the nucleus that contain DNA

_____ 12. hormone that stimulates production of gametes in men and women

_____ 13. sex cells

Section 16.1 Study Questions

1. In which cells in the body do mitosis and meiosis occur?

2. Explain the differences between mitosis and meiosis.

3. Define *haploid* and *diploid*.

4. List common chromosomal abnormalities related to nondisjunction.

5. What is the function of the SRY gene?

6. At what gestational age do males and females differentiate?

7. Describe the levels of FSH and LH in a newborn, relative to those in early childhood.

8. Which hormones bring about puberty?

9. List the changes that occur in females during puberty.

10. List the changes that occur in males during puberty.

Section 16.2 Vocabulary Review

Match each vocabulary word with its definition.

A. bulbourethral glands
B. ductus deferens
C. ejaculation
D. epididymis
E. erection
F. gonads
G. penis
H. prostate gland
I. semen
J. seminal glands
K. seminiferous tubules
L. sperm

_____ 1. duct that goes from the epididymis to the ejaculatory duct

_____ 2. contains sperm and secretions from the bulbourethral glands, prostate, and seminal glands

_____ 3. state in which the penis becomes engorged with blood

_____ 4. male sex cell

_____ 5. location of sperm maturation

_____ 6. small glands that add mucus to semen

_____ 7. delivers sperm to the female system

_____ 8. gland that surrounds the urethra and contributes to semen

_____ 9. the discharging of sperm

_____ 10. organs that produce sex cells

_____ 11. location of sperm production

_____ 12. glands that are the major contributor to semen

Section 16.2 Study Questions

1. At what temperature is sperm formation most vigorous, and how is this temperature maintained?
2. What occurs during a vasectomy and how does it prevent fertilization?
3. Where in the testes are sperm produced?
4. What is the function of the epididymis?

5. What is a hernia?
6. What occurs during a circumcision?
7. Trace the ductwork through which sperm travel.
8. What is the difference between semen and sperm?
9. Which glands contribute to semen?
10. Describe the structure of sperm and the timetable for sperm development.

Section 16.2 Labeling
Male Reproductive Organs

Identify the organs of the male reproductive system.

Labeling Terms

A. ampulla of ductus deferens
B. anus
C. bulb of penis
D. bulbourethral gland
E. corpus cavernosum
F. corpus spongiosum
G. ductus deferens (vas deferens)

H. ejaculatory duct
I. epididymis
J. external urethral orifice
K. glans penis
L. prepuce
M. prostate
N. pubis

O. rectum
P. scrotum
Q. seminal gland (seminal vesicle)
R. testis
S. ureter
T. urethra
U. urinary bladder

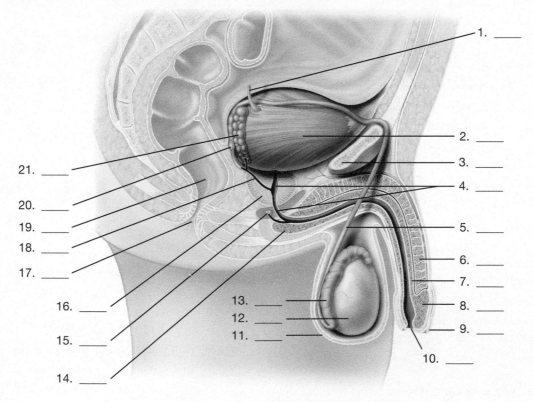

© Body Scientific International

Testis and Epididymis

Identify the structures of the testis and epididymis.

Labeling Terms

A. body of epididymis
B. blood vessels and nerves
C. ductus deferens (vas deferens)
D. head of epididymis
E. seminiferous tubule
F. spermatic cord
G. tail of epididymis
H. testis

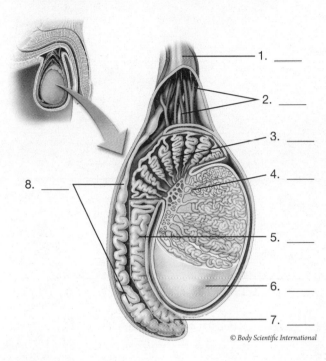

1. ____
2. ____
3. ____
4. ____
5. ____
6. ____
7. ____
8. ____

© Body Scientific International

Sperm Cell

Identify the parts of a sperm cell.

Labeling Terms

A. acrosome
B. centriole
C. flagellum
D. head
E. midpiece
F. mitochondria
G. nucleus

Sperm Cell

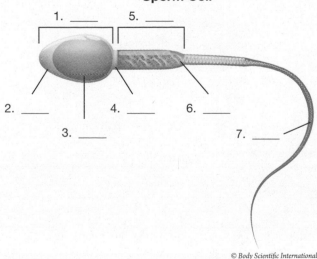

1. ____
2. ____
3. ____
4. ____
5. ____
6. ____
7. ____

© Body Scientific International

Section 16.3 Vocabulary Review

Match each vocabulary word with its definition.

A. cervix
B. clitoris
C. labia majora
D. labia minora
E. lactiferous duct
F. mammary glands
G. oocyte
H. oogenesis
I. ovarian cycle
J. ovulation
K. uterine cycle
L. uterine tubes
M. uterus
N. vagina

____ 1. innermost folds surrounding the vaginal opening
____ 2. birth canal portion inferior to the uterus
____ 3. produce milk
____ 4. process of releasing an oocyte from the ovary
____ 5. process of forming oocytes
____ 6. outermost folds surrounding the vaginal opening
____ 7. structure in which fertilization occurs
____ 8. egg cell
____ 9. bottom portion of uterus that dilates prior to delivery
____ 10. female erectile tissue
____ 11. site of implantation
____ 12. includes menstrual, proliferative, and secretory phases
____ 13. transports milk
____ 14. includes the maturation and release of an oocyte

Section 16.3 Study Questions

1. Where are ova produced, and how do they enter the uterine tube?
2. Where does fertilization normally occur? Where does implantation occur?
3. What is an ectopic pregnancy, and why is it a cause for concern?
4. Describe the layers of the uterus.
5. What female structures are classified as external genitalia?
6. Describe the ductwork in a mammary gland.
7. What is the timetable for oogenesis?
8. Describe the events that occur in the follicular phase of the ovarian cycle.
9. Describe the events that occur in the luteal phase of the ovarian cycle.
10. What changes occur in the uterine cycle?

Section 16.3 Labeling
Female Reproductive Organs

Identify the structures and organs of the female reproductive system.

Labeling Terms

A. ampulla
B. body of uterus
C. cervical canal
D. cervix
E. endometrium

F. fimbriae
G. fundus of uterus
H. infundibulum
I. isthmus
J. lumen (cavity) of uterus

K. myometrium
L. oocyte
M. ovarian blood vessels
N. ovary
O. perimetrium

P. ureter
Q. uterine blood vessels
R. uterine (fallopian) tube
S. vagina

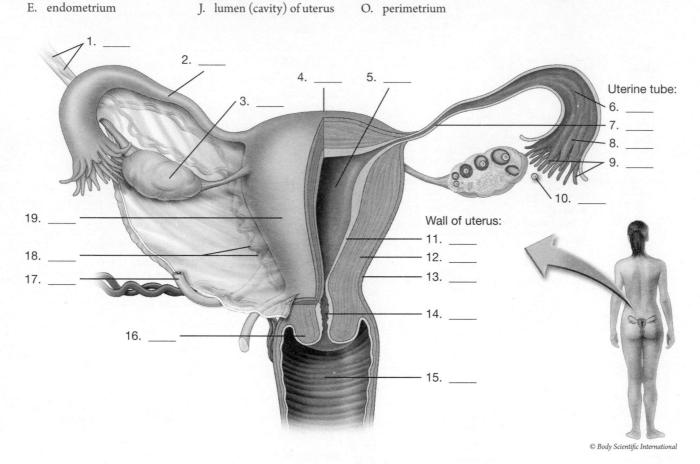

1. ____
2. ____
3. ____
4. ____
5. ____

Uterine tube:
6. ____
7. ____
8. ____
9. ____
10. ____

19. ____
18. ____
17. ____
16. ____

Wall of uterus:
11. ____
12. ____
13. ____
14. ____
15. ____

© Body Scientific International

Mammary Gland

Identify the structures of the mammary gland in the female breast.

Labeling Terms

A. adipose tissue
B. areola
C. first rib
D. hypodermis
   (superficial fascia)
E. intercostal muscles
F. lactiferous duct
G. lobe
H. lobule
I. nipple
J. opening of lactiferous duct
K. pectoralis major muscle
L. skin (cut)

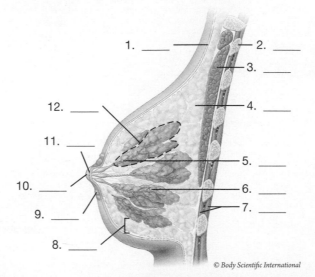

1. ____
2. ____
3. ____
4. ____
5. ____
6. ____
7. ____
8. ____
9. ____
10. ____
11. ____
12. ____

© Body Scientific International

Name: _____   Date: _____

Section 16.4 Vocabulary Review

Match each vocabulary word with its definition.

A. amniotic fluid
B. blastocyst
C. delivery of the placenta
D. dilation
E. embryo
F. expulsion
G. fetus
H. human chorionic gonadotropin (hCG)

I. implantation
J. lactation
K. letdown reflex
L. oxytocin
M. placenta
N. prolactin
O. umbilical cord

_____ 1. process in which a blastocyst connects to the endometrium

_____ 2. fluid surrounding a fetus

_____ 3. hormone that stimulates milk production

_____ 4. name for an unborn child from eight weeks after conception until birth

_____ 5. connects the fetus to the placenta

_____ 6. hormone that stimulates the placenta to make progesterone

_____ 7. name for an embryo from four to six days after fertilization

_____ 8. hormone that produces uterine contractions

_____ 9. stage of labor in which the cervical opening enlarges

_____ 10. stage of labor after the baby has been born

_____ 11. organ in the uterus that supplies the baby with nutrients

_____ 12. name for an unborn child from implantation to eighth week of gestation

_____ 13. stage of labor that ends when the baby is delivered

_____ 14. secretion of milk from the mammary glands

_____ 15. smooth muscle action in a mother that allows the baby to receive milk

Section 16.4 Study Questions

1. What does capacitation accomplish?
2. How does the sperm fertilize the oocyte?
3. What events occur to protect against polyspermy?
4. How is the duration of a pregnancy measured?
5. Explain the difference between monozygotic and dizygotic twins.
6. What is the function of human chorionic gonadotropin (hCG) in maintaining a pregnancy?
7. What is the function of the placenta?
8. Describe the events that occur in each of the three stages of labor.
9. What are the two hormones involved in milk production and secretion?
10. What is the let-down reflex, and how is it initiated?

Section 16.4 Labeling

Fetal Environment

Identify the structures that surround the fetus in the mother's uterus.

Labeling Terms

A. amnion
B. amniotic cavity
C. cervix
D. chorion
E. decidua capsularis
F. lumen of uterus
G. placenta
H. umbilical cord
I. uterus

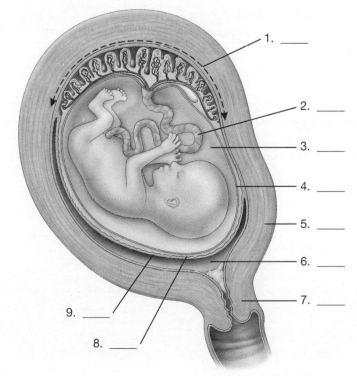

1. _____
2. _____
3. _____
4. _____
5. _____
6. _____
7. _____
8. _____
9. _____

© Body Scientific International

Section 16.5 Vocabulary Review

Match each vocabulary word with its definition.

A. chlamydia
B. genital herpes
C. gonorrhea
D. human papillomavirus (HPV)
E. infertility
F. sexually transmitted infection

_____ 1. any infection that occurs because of sexual contact

_____ 2. infection that does not always have symptoms, but can damage uterine tubes and increase the risk of ectopic pregnancy

_____ 3. causes genital warts and cervical cancer

_____ 4. inability to get pregnant

_____ 5. infection that may result in painful urination or no symptoms, but can cause infertility

_____ 6. infection that causes blistering around genital area or mouth

Section 16.5 Study Questions

1. List common causes of male infertility.
2. What are some common causes of female infertility?
3. How can infertility be treated?
4. Which is the most lethal sexually transmitted infection?
5. What results from untreated syphilis?
6. What are the symptoms of pelvic inflammatory disease?
7. What conditions occur more commonly in people who are infected with the human papillomavirus (HPV) than in people who do not have an HPV infection?
8. How is prostate cancer detected and treated?
9. What diseases are more common in women who have abnormal BRCA genes?
10. How is breast cancer detected and treated?

Medical Terminology

For each item, identify the word parts and their meanings, and then provide the meaning of the medical term. Use a medical dictionary or the textbook if you need help.

1. polydactyly

   prefix: _____

   meaning: _____

   root/combining form: _____

   meaning: _____

   suffix: _____

   meaning: _____

   meaning of word: _____

2. metrorrhagia

   root/combining form: _____

   meaning: _____

   suffix: _____

   meaning: _____

   meaning of word: _____

3. perichondrium

   prefix: _____

   meaning: _____

   root/combining form: _____

   meaning: _____

   suffix: _____

   meaning: _____

   meaning of word: _____

4. polyhydramnios

   prefix: _____

   meaning: _____

   root/combining form: _____

   meaning: _____

   root/combining form: _____

   meaning: _____

   meaning of word: _____

5. inguinal orchiectomy

   root/combining form: _____

   meaning: _____

   suffix: _____

   meaning: _____

   root/combining form: _____

   meaning: _____

   suffix: _____

   meaning: _____

   meaning of word: _____

6. polydipsia

    prefix: _____

    meaning: _____

    root/combining form: _____

    meaning: _____

    suffix: _____

    meaning: _____

    meaning of word: _____

7. perionychia

    prefix: _____

    meaning: _____

    root/combining form: _____

    meaning: _____

    suffix: _____

    meaning: _____

    meaning of word: _____

8. polymyalgia

    prefix: _____

    meaning: _____

    root/combining form: _____

    meaning: _____

    suffix: _____

    meaning: _____

    meaning of word: _____

9. periaortic

    prefix: _____

    meaning: _____

    root/combining form: _____

    meaning: _____

    suffix: _____

    meaning: _____

    meaning of word: _____

10. periarticular

    prefix: _____

    meaning: _____

    root/combining form: _____

    meaning: _____

    suffix: _____

    meaning: _____

    meaning of word: _____

NOTES

Anatomy and Physiology Word Elements

Many word parts that are routinely used in the study of anatomy and physiology come from Greek and Latin. The meanings of these word parts offer clues to the meanings of words used to describe structures, functions, and processes. For example, the word physiology is made up of physio- ("function") and -logy ("study of"). Thus, physiology is the study of how living things function or work. Likewise, the word anatomy comes from ana- ("apart") and -tomy ("cutting"). These word elements are appropriate when you consider that ancient anatomists gained a great deal of knowledge about the structure of tissues and organs through dissection.

Understanding the meanings of word parts will help you as you study anatomy and physiology.

A

ab- away from, off (*abdominal aorta, abduction*)
abdomen/o abdomen (*abdominal, abdominopelvic cavity*)
acous/o, acoust/o hearing, sound (*external acoustic meatus*)
acr/o- extremity, highest or farthest point (*acromegaly, acromion*)
ad- to, toward, near (*adduction*)
adip/o- fat or fatty tissue (*adipocyte, adipose tissue*)
af- toward (*afferent nerves, afferent pathway*)
-agon to gather, assemble (*agonist, antagonist*)
alb/i, alb/o, albin/o white (*albinism*)
amni- fetal sac (*amnion, amniotic fluid*)
amph-, amphi/o on both sides, around (*amphiarthrosis*)
an- not, without (*anaerobic, anemia*)
ana- apart (anatomy, anaphase); up, build up (*anabolism*)
andr/o male (*androgen*)
angi/o blood vessel (*angioplasty, angiography, angiotensin*)
antero forward, from front to back (*anteroposterior*)
anti- against (*antibiotic, antidiuretic hormone*)
apo- above, away, off, separated from (*apocrine glands, aponeurosis*)
aque/o water (*aquaporins, aqueous humor*)
arteri/o artery (*arterial, arterioles*)
arthr/o joint (*synarthroses, diarthrodial*)
articul/o joint (*articular fibrocartilage, articulating bones*)
-ase enzyme (*amylase, polymerase*)
ather/o fat, plaque (*atherosclerosis*)
atri/o heart, entryway (*atrium, interatrial septum*)
audi/o, audit/o hearing (*auditory canal, audiologist*)
aur/i, aur/o, auricul/o ear, hearing (*auricle*)
aut/o self (*autoimmune disease, autonomic nervous system*)
axi/o axis, straight line (*axial skeleton, axon*)

B

bar/o pressure, weight (*baroreceptors, barometric*)
bi- two, twice, double (*bicarbonate, biceps*)
bi/o life (*biopsy, microbial*)
bil/i bile (*bilirubin*)
blast/o bud, germ, precursor (*blastocyst, osteoblast*)
brachi/o arm (*biceps brachii*)
bronch/i, bronch/o airway (*bronchus, bronchodilator*)

C

calc/o, calci/o calcium, stone (*hypercalcemia, calcitonin*)
calori- heat (*Calorie, caloric*)
carcin/o cancer (*carcinogen*)
cardi/o heart (*cardiovascular*)

carp/o wrist (*metacarpals, radiocarpal*)
centr/i, centr/o middle, center (*centromere, centriole*)
cephal/o head (*diencephalon, brachiocephalic artery*)
cerebr/o brain (*cerebrum*)
cervic/o neck, narrow part (*cervical*)
circ/um- around, about (*circumduction*)
-clast break (down), destroy (*osteoclasts*)
clavicul/o hammer, club, key (*clavicle, acromioclavicular joint*)
-cle little (*corpuscle*)
co- with, together (*cotransport*)
col-, col/o, col/ono- large intestine (*colonoscopy*)
com- with, together (*complement system, compression*)
contus/o bruise (*contusion*)
coron/o heart, crown (*coronary, corona radiata*)
corp/o, corpor/o body (*corpus luteum, corpora cavernosa*)
corti- covering (*cortical*)
cost/o rib (*intercostal nerves, sternocostal joints*)
cox/a, cox/o hip (*coxal bone*)
crani/o skull (*cranium*)
-crin/o secrete, separate (*endocrine, exocrine*)
cry/o cold (*cryotherapy, oocyte cryopreservation*)
-cule, -culus small (*molecule, canaliculus*)
cutane/o skin (*subcutaneous fascia, musculocutaneous*)
cyst/i, cyst/o bladder (*cystitis, cholecystectomy*)
-cyte, cyt/o cell (*lymphocyte, cytoplasm*)

D

de- down, away from, cessation (*dehydration, defibrillation*)
dendr/o tree, branch (*dendrites, oligodendrocytes*)
-derma, dermat/o, derm/o skin (*epidermal, dermatologist*)
-desis binding, tying together (*diapedesis*)
desm/o bond, ligament (*desmosomes, syndesmosis*)
di- two, apart, separate, through (*diuresis, antidiuretic hormone*)
dia- across, separate, through (*diaphragm, dialysis*)
dif- apart, separate (*differentiate, diffusion*)
digit- finger (*extensor digitorum*)
dilat/o widening, expanding, stretching (*dilation*)
dipl/o double (*diploid*)
dis- apart, separate (*dissect, dislocation*)
dist/o far, distant (*distal convoluted tubule*)
dors/i, dors/o back, back of body (*dorsal, latissimus dorsi*)
duc-, duct/o to lead, carry (*abduction, adduction*)
dynam/o strength, force, power, energy (*dynamic lung volume, dynamometer*)
dys- bad, abnormal, painful (*muscular dystrophy, dyspnea*)

E

e- out (*ejaculate, eversion*)

-eal pertaining to (*pineal, esophageal*)

ec-, ect/o out, outside, away (*ectopic*)

-ectomy incision, surgical removal (*cholecystectomy, mastectomy*)

-edema swelling (*lymphedema, myxedema*)

ef- out, out of (*efferent, effusion*)

-el, -elle small (*organelle, fontanel*)

electr/o electricity (*electrocardiogram, electrolytes*)

em- in, within (*embolism*)

-ema condition (*emphysema*)

-emia blood condition (*anemia, leukemia*)

en- in, into (*enzyme*)

encephal/o brain (*diencephalon*)

end/o in, inside, within (*endometrium*)

enter/o intestine (*gastroenterologist*)

epi- on, upon, above (*epidermis, epididymis*)

epitheli/o skin (*epithelium*)

erythr/o red (*erythrocyte*)

-esis action, condition, state of (*erythropoiesis, synthesis*)

estr/o female (*estrogen*)

ex-, exo- out, out of, away, away from (*exocytosis, exophthalmos*)

extra- outside (*extracellular*)

F

femor/o thigh bone (*femoral*)

fer-, -ferent to carry (*afferent, efferent*)

fibr/o fiber (*fibroblast*)

fil/a, fil/o, filament/o thread, thread-like (*microfilament, filtration*)

flex/o bend (*dorsiflexion*)

fore- before (*forearm*); in front (*forehead*)

-form, -iform having the shape or form of (*fusiform, deformed*)

G

gastr/o stomach (*gastric, gastroesophageal*)

-gen, -genic, -genesis producing, bringing about (*gluconeogenesis, oogenesis*)

germi- sprout, bud (*germinate, germinal*)

gest/o to carry (*ingest*); pregnancy (*gestation, progesterone*)

gingiv/o pertaining to the gums (*gingivitis*)

glauc/o having a blue or blue-gray color (*glaucoma*)

-glia glue (*neuroglia, microglia*)

globu- sphere, ball (*globulin, hemoglobin*)

gloss/o, glott/o tongue (*glossopharyngeal*)

gluc/o sugar, glucose (*glucose, glucocorticoid*)

glyc/o sugar, glucose (*glycogen, hypoglycemia, glycolysis*)

-gnosis knowledge (*diagnosis, prognosis*)

gon/o, gonad/o semen, seed, pertaining to reproduction (*spermatogonia, gonadotropic*)

gyn/o, gynec/o woman, female (*gynecology*)

H

hapl/o single, simple (*haploid*)

hema-, hemo-, hemat/o blood (*hematopoiesis, hematocrit*)

hemi- half (*hemisphere*)

-hemia blood condition (*polycythemia*)

hepat/o liver (*hepatitis*)

hist/o tissue (*histology*)

hom/o like, similar (*homologous*)

home/o unchanging, constant (*homeostasis*)

humer/o shoulder (*humerus*)

hydr/o water (*hydrophobic*)

hyper- above, above normal, excessive (*hypertrophy, hyperopia*)

hypo- under, below normal (*hypoxia, hyposecretion*)

I

-ia condition (*anemia, pneumonia*)

-iasis abnormal condition (*psoriasis*)

-iatr/o doctor, medicine (*pediatric*)

-ic, -ical pertaining to (*anatomical, biological*)

-icle, -icul small (*ossicle, canaliculus*)

-ics knowledge (*kinetics, genetics*)

-immun/o protection, safety (*autoimmune, immunotherapy*)

in- in, into, not (*inspiration*)

-in(e) protein, enzyme, chemical compound (*penicillin, creatinine*)

infra- below, beneath, inferior to (*infraspinous fossa*)

inter- between, among (*interstitial, intervertebral*)

intra- within, into (*intracellular*)

-ism process (*metabolism*); condition or disorder (*gigantism, astigmatism*)

is/o same, equal (*isometric*)

-ite little (*dendrite*)

-itis inflammation (*gingivitis*)

-ium structure, tissue (*cranium, endomysium*)

J

jaund/o yellow (*jaundice*)

jug- to join (*jugular*)

juxta- beside, next to (*juxtamedullary nephrons*)

K

kerat/o hard, horn-shaped tissue (*keratinocytes*)

kin/e, kin/o, kines/o, kinesi/o movement, motion (*kinetic, cytokinesis*)

L

lacrim/o tear (*lacrimal glands*)

lact/i, lact/o milk (*lactation*)

laryng/o voice box (*laryngeal*)

later/o side (*lateral rotation*)

-lepsy, -leptic seizure (*epilepsy, epileptic*)

-let small (*platelet*)

leuk/o white (*leukocytes, leukemia*)

lig/o to tie, bind (*ligament*)

lingu/a, lingu/o tongue (*lingual tonsil*)

lip/o fat (*lipocyte*)

lith/o stone (*lithotripsy*)

-(o)logy study of (*biology, physiology*)

-lucent, -lucid clear, light, shining (*zona pellucida, stratum lucidum*)

lumb/o lower back (*lumbar*)

lun- moon, crescent (*semilunar valves*)

lute/o yellow (*corpus luteum*)

-lymph, lymph/o lymph (*endolymph, lymphocytes*)

lys/o, lyt/o, -lyt/ic separate, break apart, break down, destroy (*lysosome, glycolysis*)

M

macro- large (*macrophage*)

mal/i bad (*malfunction, malignant*)

mamm/o breast (*mammogram*)

medi/o, mediastin/o middle (*medial, mediastinum*)

medull/o middle, deep part, marrow (*medullary canal, medulla oblongata*)

meg/a, megal/o, -megaly large, enlargement (*acromegaly, megakaryocytes*)

melan/o black color (*melanocyte, melanoma*)

men/o month, menses, menstruation (*amenorrhea, menarche*)

mening/o, meningi/o membrane (*meningitis*)

meta- after, beyond; change (*metaphase, metacarpal*)

-meter instrument or device used to measure (*spirometer, sphygmomanometer*)

metri- length, measure (*metric system*)

metri-, metr/o uterus, womb (*endometrium*)

micro- small; millionth (*microscope, microbiology*)

mon/o one, single (*monomer, monosaccharide*)

morph/o form, shape (*polymorphism*)

-mortem, mort/o death (*mortality, postmortem*)

muc/o, mucos/o mucus (*mucosal*)

multi- many (*multicellular*)

muscul/o muscle (*musculoskeletal*)

muta- change (*mutation*)

myel/o bone marrow (*myeloid*); spinal cord (*myelin*)

mysi-, my/o, myos/o muscle (*myositis, epimysium*)

N

nas/o nose (*nasolacrimal, nasopharynx*)

natr/i, natr/o sodium (*hyponatremia, natriuretic*)

neo- new (*gluconeogenesis, neonatal*)

nephr/o kidney (*nephron*)

neur/o nerve (*neuromuscular, neuroscience*)

neutr/o neutral, neither (*neutrophil, neutralization*)

nucle/o nucleus (*nuclear membrane, deoxyribonucleic acid*)

nutri/o, nutrit/o nourish (*nutrient, nutrition*)

O

obstetr/o pregnancy; birth (*obstetrician*)

ocul/o eye (*oculomotor, orbicularis oculi*)

odont/o tooth (*periodontal disease*)

-ole little, small (*arteriole, nucleolus*)

-oma tumor, mass (*carcinoma, hematoma*)

onc/o tumor (*oncologist*)

-opia vision condition (*myopia, hyperopia*)

ophthalm/o eye (*ophthalmologist, exophthalmos*)

-opsy view of (*biopsy*)

optic/o eye, vision (*optic chiasma*)

or/o mouth (*oropharynx*)

orbi- circle (*orbicularis*)

-orexia appetite (*anorexia*)

orth/o straight (*orthopedic, orthodontist*)

-ose sugar (*glucose, fructose*)

-osis process (*mitosis, apoptosis*); disease, abnormal condition (*tuberculosis, cirrhosis*)

osseo- bony (*osseous tissue, interosseous membrane*)

ossi- bone (*ossification*)

ost/e, oste/o bone (*osteoporosis*)

ov/o, ovul/o egg (*ovum, ovulation*)

ox/o oxygen (*hypoxic, oxyhemoglobin*)

P

para- near, next to, beside (*parathyroid, parasites*)

-partum birth; labor (*parturition, postpartum*)

path/o disease (*pathology*); feeling, emotion (*sympathetic*)

pector/o chest (*pectoral girdle, pectoralis major*)

ped/o child (*pediatrician*); foot (*tinea pedis*)

pelv/i, pelv/o hip (*pelvic*)

pend/o to hang (*appendix, appendicular*)

-penia deficiency (*osteopenia*)

penna- thread (*unipennate*)

penta- five, fifth (*pentapeptide, pentamer*)

peri- around (*periosteum, peritoneum*)

-phage, phag/o eat, swallow (*esophagus, phagocytosis*)

phalang/o fingers, toes (*phalanges*)

pharyng/o throat (*pharyngeal*)

phil/o loving, attracted to (*hydrophilic*)

phleb/o vein (*phlebotomist*)

-phob/o, -phobia fear (*hydrophobic*)

phon/o, -phonia voice, sound (*phonetic*)

phot/o light (*phototherapy*)

physi/o, physic/o nature, function (*physiology, physician*)

-physis growth (*diaphysis, epiphysis*)

-plasm shaped, molded (*cytoplasm, endoplasmic*)

-plasty surgical repair (*rhinoplasty*)

-plegia, -plegic paralysis (*paraplegia*)

pleur/o lung (*pleurisy*)

plex/o network of nerves (*brachial plexus*)

-pnea breath, breathing (*dyspnea*)

pneum/o, pneumon/o lung, air (*pneumonia*)

pod/o foot (*podocyte*)

-poiesis formation (*hematopoiesis, erythropoiesis*)

-poietin substance that forms (*erythropoietin, thrombopoietin*)

poly- many, much (*polymer, polysaccharide*)

-porosis condition of holes, spaces (*osteoporosis*)

post- after, behind (*postmenopausal*)

poster/o back of (the body), behind (*posterior*)

pre- before, in front of (*precursor, preganglionic*)

presby/o old age (*presbyopia*)

pro- before, in front of (*prostate*); promote (*progesterone*)

prot/o first (*protoplasm*)

proxim/o near (*proximal*)

pseudo false (*pseudopod*)

psych/o mind (*psychological*)

pulmon/o lung (*pulmonary*)

puls/o, pulsat/o to beat, vibrate, push against (*pulsation, propulsion*)

pyr/o, pyret/o, pyrex/o fire; fever (*pyrogen*)

Q

quadri- four (*quadriceps*)
quater- fourth (*quaternary structure*)

R

radiat- radiating (*corona radiata*)
radi/o X-ray; radioactive (*radiography*)
re- back, again, backward (*reabsorption, remodeling*)
-receptor, -ceptor receiver (*chemoreceptor*)
ren/o kidney (*renal cortex*)
respir/o breathe (*respiratory*)
reticul/o network (*reticular connective tissue*)
retr/o back, backward, behind (*retroperitoneal*)
rhin/o nose (*rhinoplasty*)
-rrhage, -rrhagia bursting forth of blood (*hemorrhagic stroke*)
-rrhea flow, discharge (*diarrhea, amenorrhea*)

S

sacchar/o sugar (*polysaccharide*)
sacr/o posterior section of pelvic bone (*sacroiliac joint*)
scapul/o shoulder blade (*scapulothoracic joint, subscapular*)
-scope, scop/o, -scopy see (*microscope, colonoscope*)
sect/o to cut (*dissection*)
semi- half (*semicircular canals, semilunar valves*)
semin/i semen, seed (*seminal glands, seminiferous tubules*)
-sis state of, condition (*stenosis*); process (*mitosis, glycolysis*)
son/o sound (*sonogram*)
-spasm sudden contraction of muscles (*bronchospasm*)
sperm/o, spermat/o sperm cells (*spermatid, spermatocyte*)
-sphyxia pulse (*asphyxiation*)
spir/o to breathe (*respiration, spirometer*)
stas/i, stat/i stop, remain, stay the same (*homeostasis*)
-static pertaining to stopping or controlling (*homeostatic, hydrostatic*)
sten/o narrow, constricted (*valvular stenosis*)
stern/o chest, breast (*sternum*)
steth/o chest (*stethoscope*)
strept/o twisted chains (*streptococcus*)
stri/a striped (*striated*)
sub- under, below (*subcutaneous*)
super- above, beyond (*superior, superficial*)
sym- together, with (*symphysis, symmetrical*)
syn- together, with (*synthesis, synarthroses*)
synaps/o, synapt/o to join, make contact (*synaptic*)
systol/o contraction (*systolic*)

T

tars/i, tars/o ankle, hindfoot (*metatarsal*)
tendin/o, ten/o tendon (*tendinitis*)
tens/o stretched, strained (*tensile*)
tetra- four (*tetramer, tetrad*)
therm/o heat (*hyperthermia, thermometer*)
thorac/o, -thorax chest, pleural cavity (*cardiothoracic*)
thromb/o blood clot (*thrombosis, thrombocytes*)
tom/o to cut (*splenectomy, cholecystectomy*)
tox/o, toxic/o poison (*cytotoxic*)
trans- across, through (*neurotransmitter, transverse plane*)
tri- three (*adenosine triphosphate, triglycerides*)
-tropin to act on, stimulate (*adrenocorticotropin, gonadotropin*)

U

-ul, -ule little, small (*trabecula, glomerulus*)
ultra- beyond, excessive (*ultraviolet, ultrasonic*)
-um structure, tissue, substance (*cerebrum, sodium*)
uni- one (*unipennate, unipolar*)
-uresis urination (*diuresis*)
ur/i, ur/o, -uria, urin/o urine, urination (*polyuria, urinalysis*)
-us structure, thing (*fetus, hypothalamus*)
uter/o womb (*uterus, uterine*)

V

valv/o, valvu/o valve (*valvular stenosis*)
vas/o, vascul/o vessel (*vasa recta, vascular, vas deferens*)
ven/i, ven/o vein (*venous, venule, intravenous*)
ventil/o to oxygenate (*ventilation, hyperventilation*)
ventr/o, ventricul/o belly side of body, lower part (*ventral, ventricle*)
vers/o, -verse, -version turning (*eversion, inversion*)
vertebr/o spine; backbone (*intervertebral*)
vir/o virus (*viral, virology*)
viscer/o internal organs (*visceral pleura, visceral pericardium*)
vit/a, vit/o life (*vitamin, vital signs*)
vitr/e, vitr/o glass (*vitreous humor, in vitro*)

X

xanth/o yellow (*xanthosis*)
xiph/o sword-shaped (*xiphoid process*)

Y

-y condition, process (*thermoplasty*)

Z

zo/o life (*zoology*)
zyg/o union, junction, pair (*zygote*)